HOLISTIC PTSD RECOVERY

FOR FIRST RESPONDERS, MILITARY & THEIR FAMILIES

BY SARAH K. GRACE

Gratitude to Rachel Koontz, Jessa Mohaddess, Kat Lusher, Svanhild Simonson and Nick Shuster for your diligent support in bringing this book to completion. I couldn't have done it without you. And for my amazing children, Ava and Aidan, who inspire me to be the best I can be every day.

Stronger Together.

The stories in this book are compilations of personal experience provided by actual individuals. Some of the names and details have been changed, modified, or fictionalized in order to protect privacy. While I acknowledge that military personnel and first responders differ, I also understand that there are enough similarities to include all branches of service together in this book. I honor ALL front line workers and service personnel. Thank you for all that you do.

Disclaimer:

I am not a doctor. All modalities listed are suggestions. I do not advocate any specific therapy and cannot be held liable for your choices, experiences or actions. If you choose to engage in any or all of the following modalities, I recommend you have the support of a therapist, healer, and/or doctor to assist your process. Do not try to do this alone. Significant discomfort can result from embarking on the healing journey. You are ultimately responsible for your own wellbeing, choices, and actions and outcome.

TABLE OF CONTENTS

My Story

It was a sunny Sunday morning as my veteran EMT partner Rob and I dropped off a patient at the local hospital. A routine transfer, our patient was a pleasant eighty-three-year-old woman who required further tests for her heart condition. After giving the dark-haired nurse a turnover report, I slowly returned to the ambulance to complete my paperwork.

"I'm hungry and I need some coffee," Rob said to me. "Can you finish that paperwork on a drive over to Starbucks?"

"Sure," I said. "That actually sounds good. I could use some caffeine too."

Jumping in, we notified dispatch and pulled out of the hospital bay, turning left onto the busy street.

Nonchalantly tapping the steering wheel with his hands, Rob said, "I pulled some overtime and am on the homestretch of a thirty six hour shift. I can't wait to get home and see my baby boy. He turns six months old tomorrow."

"Congratulations!" I said. "Thirty six hours, eh? I'll bet you'll be glad to get out of here."

"Yeah. It's been a long one. We didn't have anything too crazy though... so that's good."

Pulling into the Starbucks parking lot, Rob and I noticed a woman in her mid-thirties walking briskly down the sidewalk toward an adjacent gas station. Petite with sandy blonde hair, she was talking loudly to herself and making angry gestures toward the sky. "Is she?" Rob started. "Yup. She's talking to herself," I said. Knowing there was a psychiatric facility a few blocks away Rob said, "Maybe she was discharged this morning..." "Maybe," I said. "Let's hope she's still on her meds..."

The woman went inside the gas station and appeared to be talking to the attendant.

"He's probably going to call 911 and we'll end up responding over there," Rob said, "Quick, let's get our coffee before he does."

We had just enough time to order, make a bathroom stop, and walk back to the ambulance before dispatch notified us to respond to the gas station. "Copy that, you can mark us arriving first on scene." Rob replied. While driving across the street, we watched the blonde-haired woman walk back outside the station and hunch over by one of the gas pumps.

"What is she doing?" I said.

"I don't know…" Rob replied curiously.

In what seemed like a split second, the woman lifted a container and started pouring gasoline all over herself. "What the…?" but before I could even get the words out, we saw the spark of a lighter in her hand.

"Oh shit…" Rob said.

Everything stopped. All noise from the city ceased. Birds froze midair. Cars no longer moved. There was a deafening silence that somehow pulled me forward, like I was being sucked into a black hole. My body felt hot. I tasted metal. From where she stood, the woman's troubled blue eyes locked onto mine and I could feel her pain. I knew we were about to watch her die, and because it all happened so fast, there was little we could do.

With a 'whoosh' the petite woman became a blazing inferno. Rob and I froze, watching a flailing, screaming ball of fire run around in circles away from the gas pumps and toward the front of our ambulance. The smell of burnt hair and flesh wafted over us as the shrill shrieks of hysteria and agony filled our ears. I put my hand on the door to get out, but Rob stopped me. "You can't." he said. "First rule of EMS – don't become a patient yourself. She might try to grab onto you. We have to extinguish her first."

Nauseated, I grabbed the radio, "Dispatch, we need PD and an engine to our location Code 3. Hurry!" "Copy that," dispatch replied, "Engine 10 has a four-minute ETA." Our ambulance only had one little fire extinguisher, not nearly enough to put her out. So we watched, and waited. Helpless. Silent. Listening to her screams growing softer, and her flailing circles getting smaller. At one point the burning ball stopped and slowly turned toward us, the skin from her face dripping down and hanging off her skull like melted wax, black sockets in the place where her blue eyes had just been.

"Oh my God," I whispered.

Minutes that felt like years passed and finally Engine 10 arrived. Frantic, muffled voices came from somewhere far away, yelling at each other to pull the hose. Water doused in slow motion. I watched the crystalline droplets hit her burning flesh. Her shrieks became whimpers. Her whimpers became silence. I heard nothing but my breath. Finally, the flames went out and her charred body fell into a tiny, smoldering pile on the sidewalk in front of our ambulance.

■

My name is Sarah K. Grace. I've been a licensed paramedic and holistic healing practitioner in California for nearly twenty years. My 911 career began in the Compton/Inglewood areas of South Central LA before moving on to San Jose and Sacramento. In addition to field time, I've taught paramedic school and proctored National Registry exams for fifteen years. Beyond western medicine, I've also studied holistic healing in the forms of reiki, shamanism, medical intuition, and energy healing for many years. My first book, *Journey Into Grace*, is a best-seller in its genre, and I now have a thriving practice blending western medicine with energy medicine to help people all over the world overcome trauma, addiction, and PTSD.

While there are plenty of PTSD resources available, I've noticed that many are written by people who have never actually been on the front lines. I truly believe they mean well, but many military personnel and first responders have a hard time relating unless the advisor has actually been there. It's like the old saying: **It takes one to know one**. Unless someone actually knows the sights, sounds, and smells, can they truly understand?

Personally, **I didn't even realize that I had PTSD** until I developed a seriously negative attitude about people and the world in general. It crept up on me slowly, little by little over the years. At the beginning of my field time, I was always happy and upbeat—treating each day on the ambulance like an epic adventure. Stoked to be working in such a busy 911 system, I ran calls day and night. Viewing each response like a puzzle that needed to be solved as fast and efficiently as possible, the pressure and challenge lit me up. Part of me loved not knowing where I would go or what we would encounter each day. I was like a kid in a candy store. Being a paramedic was a major achievement in my life. After years of floundering, my family was finally proud of me and I was using my skills and abilities to make a difference and save lives.

But then I blinked and nearly two decades flew by. Everything had slowly changed. Where I had once been excited to go to work, I now just wanted to get my shift over with. In a perpetual state of low-grade irritation, I kept to myself more and more and my tolerance for BS calls almost completely evaporated. The curiosity and anticipation I once had were replaced by apathy and dismissal. When I used to lend a compassionate ear to patients, I now offered silence. Thousands of 911 calls under my belt and my eyes had seen too much: dead babies, drunk drivers wiping out entire families, close range shotgun blasts to the head, GI bleeds, stabbings, psychotic breaks, hangings, meth, oxy, fentanyl overdoses, eight hundred pound shut-ins, heart attacks, gang bangers, decapitations, drug seekers, decomposed bodies, homeless encampments and skid row.

What traumatized me the most wasn't what I saw, it was what I heard, smelled, and felt on calls: the sound of a mother screaming, the putrid smells of bodies burning or decomposing, the anger and hatred directed at us by patients and family members, the pressure and impatience from doctors and nurses, and the seemingly never-ending darkness of an overloaded system.

It slowly got to be too much, but the funny thing was that I didn't even realize it. My symptoms were slow and stealthy during the initial stages, almost undetectable until I developed a pessimistic attitude and significant distain for humanity. The dark things people did to one another ate away at me. Off duty, I changed, too. I was snappy with my family. When I was home, I couldn't stop thinking about work. At work, all I thought about was being home. I was never present. I started sleeping a lot and eating very little. I over-exercised and pushed my body to extremes. Nightmares and flashbacks of bad calls haunted me, so I danced with addictions to tobacco and prescription pills. When my marriage ended, things took a turn for the worse and I knew I needed help. Regular counseling didn't seem to work for me, so instead I looked into holistic healing options. Because I've always been extremely sensitive to energy, the alternative healing world seemed like a good fit.

At first, I had no idea where to start. There was no guidebook or resource telling me what to do, so I just winged it. I tried anything that sounded interesting. Some modalities worked, others didn't. But I kept at it, knowing that anything was better than where I was headed if I didn't help myself. Over time, I started noticing small changes. I became less angry and more stable. Realizing that it was important for me to get away from the toxic energy of the 911 system long enough to really get a grip, I cut back my hours on the ambulance and taught more at the paramedic school. That bit of distance helped. The better I felt, the more inspired I became to heal myself. Now I understand that everything I've ever done has led me to where I am today:

I am writing this book to help you out of the same mess I was once in myself.

The Way We Are

"First responders are like addicts going from call to call, hoping to get their fix... But over time the rush gets harder and harder to get, until eventually there's nothing left there at all."

- Bill, Fire Captain

First responders are a unique breed. We are typically hard working, blue-collar, real world people who are prone to intensity, have a twisted sense of humor, and often have a run-toward-the-fight attitude. What most of society recoils from, we find clinically fascinating. Our ability to navigate extreme volatility allows us to do our jobs but can also isolate us from others. Most of us also genuinely want to help people—often risking our lives and wellbeing to do so. Whether in military combat, running medical aids, or responding to a building collapse, our brains are wired to go *toward* the catastrophe.

So, why is that? What draws us to the crisis?

While personality types and testosterone levels certainly play a role, one often overlooked and little discussed factor in our field is that for many military personnel and first responders: **chaos is normal**. My research and personal experience suggest that many front-line workers come from very volatile backgrounds. While not everyone fits this description, those that do often have family histories of violence, addiction, impossible standards, lack of acceptance or abandonment. Many of us didn't feel safe, understood, or as though we had to prove ourselves growing up. Many of us come from a long line of military or service providers and feel compelled to carry on the family legacy. These dynamics often leads us to becoming fiercely self-reliant and able to adapt to ever-changing situations.

This 'suck it up' mentality may work on the job, but can eventually develop into a stubborn need to always be right and in control. While these traits can be good in combat or on critical 911 scenes, they often get in the way of forming close relationships.

It's a perfect recipe! Type-A personality plus unstable youth times subconscious familiarity to chaos and voila! The first responder archetype is born. Left unchecked, we often become the people who rescue others while neglecting ourselves. This common model simply works until it doesn't. Just like compensated shock, our bodies and psyches can only hold on until they can't any longer. More and more active-duty military, veterans, and first responders have hit critical mass… with addiction and suicide being the result.

Here are some other ways I've noticed first responders and military personnel differ from the mainstream crowd. As always, take what resonates and let go of what doesn't:

First responders are often adrenaline junkies.
Always on edge, many of us can never seem to relax as we await the next crisis. Our bodies and minds are always 'on.' We often develop irregular sleep patterns and can become chronically fatigued from perpetual cortisol flowing through our systems. We feel purposeful while responding to emergencies and then often crash after the call – only to repeat the cycle as we are dispatched or deployed again, and again, and

again. This high/low adrenaline cycle confuses our bodies. It can wreak havoc on our nerves, GI and endocrine systems. As a result, we can become depleted, depressed, anxious, moody, erratic or edgy.

We often look outside of ourselves for intensity.

Not satisfied with the mundane, many of us like to push our edge. This can show up in our lives through activities like combat sports, skydiving, motorcycle racing, shooting guns, working endless overtime, or even having extramarital affairs. The desire for intensity might make us feel alive for a moment, but can be destructive to our bodies, minds, and relationships.

We tend to be aggressive.

As part of a unit we still have to be able to handle our own. A crew or platoon is only as strong as their weakest link, so the group often tests and hazes each other relentlessly. This 'prove that you belong' message can be brutal, but it also establishes trust. That trust is necessary in the life-and-death circumstances that we may face together. The constant pressure to perform and be 'up to task' can be exhausting and can trigger PTSD in many forms.

We become addicted to the job.

Being a first responder or military operative is more than just work - it is an entire identity. We experience the worst aspects of humanity together. We train, live, do tours and run calls together. We fight in the trenches, endure endless hours of staging and boredom together. Sometimes, we even fight and die together. The bond between a crew, squad, platoon, or unit is indescribable to the outside world. When we are actively engaged, our identity is virtually indestructible. We are deeply connected, knowing our role and exactly how to execute. We are tapped into a lineage that flows back generations and provides us with a solid sense of purpose, structure, and power.

We are always gone.

Long tours and deployment test our relationships. From a forty-eight hour shift to six month (or longer) deployments… There is a distance from 'normal life' when on duty. Operating in a different mode, first responders do what needs to be done during the long hours at the station, on base, or in combat zones. Upon arriving home after extended time, we may be disconnected from our families and life to the point that we may even feel like a stranger in our own home. Life has a funny way of moving on while we are away, and we might just return to feel like we no longer belong. This can be challenging to all involved for obvious reasons.

We often don't know who we are without our job/role/rank.

Loss of identity through retirement, discharge, or debilitation can devastate us. Out of a powerful sense of belonging, we are suddenly faced with the question: Who am I if not this? To make the situation worse, we often feel cut off or alienated when we leave active duty. Doing what we were trained to do made us feel purposeful. Losing that strong sense of connection can be incredibly disorientating. Disconnection compounds the isolation and loss, and we can become demoralized. Many cannot cope with this abrupt end of identity or support and it may push them over the edge.

We tend to be overly Alpha.

Lastly, the intense sexual charge that frequently permeates the field is worth mentioning. Perhaps due to the hyper-masculine energy, adrenaline and risk seeking behaviors, life or death circumstances, close quarters, or a combination – sexual charge is rife among first responders and the military. This bears mention because unregulated sexual energy can be destructive when we don't know how to handle it. Unchecked, we might put ourselves in risky or destructive situations. Harassment, rape, and chain affairs are common as a result. Needless to say, these can also cause PTSD in a myriad of ways.

Take a minute to think about which of those categories. What rings true for you? What doesn't? Can you think of any other ways we differ that aren't mentioned?

In order to heal ourselves, we must first understand and accept that we tend to be different than the mainstream personality type. We think, act, and talk differently. We might be considered 'too intense, morbid, aggressive or weird' by people who have never been on the front lines. It can be hard for us to relate to the regular world when we are off duty. Family reunions, kids' birthday parties, and everyday errands can seem foreign when we've just returned from a long deployment or responded to a gruesome car wreck. Additionally, we can feel awkward around civilians. I'll never forget back when my kids were little and I took them to a park just around the corner from our house. All the other moms were busy talking about nannies and pedicures but all I could think of were the nine deaths in my response area from the latest bad batch of heroin…

Please hear me when I say that **there is nothing wrong with you**. You are part of a community of people who live beyond the mainstream construct. Your history, background, training, and career have allowed you to be of service, on-duty, during deployments, crisis and war. The fact that the mainstream day-to-day might not necessarily 'fit' once you've gone through all that is understandable.

That said, I'm here to reflect that you have the choice and ability to move beyond your training and trauma into the possibilities of a healthy new future. You can have a happy and successful life both during and after EMS and/or the military. Keeping yourself balanced during and after your career may not be easy, but as one who has healed herself from job related PTSD, I will tell you it's **worth it!**

Symptoms & Triggers

"Besides my insomnia, bulging discs, high blood pressure and chronic anxiety, I'm fine. Really. Stress is part of the job. Mainly, I cope by drinking."

- Mike, Paramedic

Jim's Story

Jim was a senior homicide detective in Detroit. Seemingly always on-call, he put in an average of eighty hours or more into work every week. With new murders almost daily, he and his colleagues did the very best they could just to keep up with the overwhelming caseload. Perpetually glued to his phone and computer, Jim was married to the job. He even frequently slept in his car or at the office just to cut down on time away from his cases. Once fresh faced and fiercely determined, twenty-five years of long hours, grizzly scenes, and agency restructuring had worn him down. As time went on his passion for exercise was replaced with sitting in an office chair for hours on end. His weight ballooned from 185 to 250 pounds, which, much to his chagrin, forced him to buy a whole new 'big sized' wardrobe. Unable to remember the last time he ate anything but fast food, Jim also developed high blood pressure and Type II diabetes. He was supposed to take medications twice a day, but only took them when he remembered.

While his health slowly spiraled, what really devastated Jim was his divorce. The relationship with the love of his life ended some years earlier because she could no longer tolerate his absence from their marriage. At the beginning, Becky had been his rock. She believed in him whole-heartedly and honestly thought that she could handle being with a man who was so devoted to his work. A sturdy woman with a mind of her own, she was extremely proud when he was promoted to detective, even beaming at him through the ceremony. But as the years passed, Jim's absence grew to be too much for her. That, and his drinking. On the rare occasion he was home, Jim routinely drank to the point of blackout.

Becky spent years pleading with Jim to get help. She tried hard, suggesting everything she could think of:

couples counseling, self-help books, AA and Al-Anon meetings. But Jim just didn't seem interested. The atrocities he saw every day had begun to bury him. Depressed, he coped by drinking booze and eating junk food. Jim had disconnected entirely from his body and emotions. Living in a hollow state of numbness, he didn't want to burden Becky with what he was going through. Justifying to himself that shutting her out was better than telling her the gruesome details, he pushed her further and further away. What was he going to say, anyway? Tell her about the three-year-old boy who was drowned in the bathtub by his bipolar mother then thrown in a back alley dumpster? Or about the beautiful twenty-two-year-old woman with her whole life ahead of her who was raped and beaten to death by her estranged boyfriend? No. Jim wanted to protect Becky, so instead of opening up to her, he locked himself in the bathroom and drank himself into oblivion.

One summer morning Jim came home from work to find divorce papers on the kitchen counter. Becky was gone. He coped with the split by drinking even more heavily and taking on bigger cases at work. From that point on he virtually lived the job. Time passed and he kept his head down and workload high. While combing through details of a local serial killer case at his desk one day, he developed a terrible headache and numbness in his left arm. Chalking it up to stress, Jim shrugged it off. That was the last thing he remembered before waking up in the hospital three days later. A doctor told him flatly that he had suffered a major stroke and was lucky to be alive. She relayed that physical therapy could potentially help him regain some of the use of his arm and leg, but that he would likely never speak normally again.

Jim knew at that moment that his career was over.

Lying alone in his hospital bed, he stared at the ceiling and listened to the stale beeping of the heart monitor. A small flower arrangement sent by a few colleagues sat on the window ledge next to a brightly colored 'Get Well Soon' card. His boss came by from admin to check on him. That was nice, but somehow none of it seemed to matter. Life as he knew it was over. Everything he had worked for over the span of nearly three decades was gone and he felt like it had all been for nothing. The heaviness of that realization crushed him. He looked down at his blank ring finger and let out a long, slow exhale.

■

PTSD has become a trendy buzzword, but what exactly is it? Technically, it's *the development of significant symptoms resulting from trauma that last two or more weeks and negatively impact daily life.* When I first read that description I thought, 'Well, that pretty much sums up every first responder ever.' But everyone handles stress differently. By nature we can manage a lot of pressure - but when we finally do reach critical mass many of us develop symptoms that can ultimately derail our lives and careers.

It's important to note that there is no one sized fits all PTSD description. Everyone is different and experiences symptoms in their own way. What might be mild PTSD for one person may be extreme for another, so it's not easy to compare. People with PTSD might have one, a few, or even all of the symptoms listed on the next page. What's important is to start paying attention to how your symptoms affect your everyday life.

In order for PTSD to be clinically diagnosed, symptoms must last longer than two weeks and have a significant impact on your daily life.

It is important to note that not everyone living with PTSD receives a diagnosis – especially those on the front lines who may resist diagnosis due to stigma. Just know that when symptoms start spilling over into everyday life and you find yourself coping, compensating or avoiding – it's time to take action to help yourself.

Below are the 30 most commonly reported symptoms of PTSD. How many do you have? How long have you had them?

☐ Anxiety	☐ Nightmares
☐ Survivor's Guilt	☐ Intrusive Memories
☐ Apathy or lack of caring about much of anything	☐ Isolation, withdrawal from close relationships
☐ Food issues: eating too much or too little	☐ Sleep issues: too much or too little
☐ Loss of motivation, Depression	☐ Dark or violent thoughts
☐ Compulsive behaviors	☐ Communication problems
☐ Explosive anger or rages	☐ Short term memory loss
☐ Negative self-image	☐ Negative world view
☐ Poor concentration	☐ Poor Judgment
☐ Flashbacks	☐ Startle Response
☐ Hypervigilance	☐ Mistrust
☐ Poor self-esteem	☐ Suicidal ideations
☐ Irritability	☐ Frustration
☐ Avoiding things that remind you of the trauma	☐ Disassociation, lack of feelings, or emotional numbness
☐ Chronic pain: ulcers, arthritis, migraines	☐ Hidden addictions: drugs, sex, or gambling

There are some schools of thought out there that say you have to cope with your symptoms forever. Personally, I don't buy that. Limping along for the rest of my life just managing symptoms doesn't really work for me. I'd rather do whatever needs to be done to heal at the root level and get on with my life in a great new way. But that's just me. It hasn't necessarily been fun, easy, or enjoyable... in fact, healing myself has been one of the most challenging (and rewarding) things I've ever done. But my nature is intense and I'd rather deal with discomfort for a shorter period of time than an entire lifetime of suffering.

What about you? Do you have symptoms of PTSD? How do they affect your life? Are you willing to be uncomfortable now to change the rest of your life for the better?

"The more you know about your personal version of PTSD, the easier it will be to know your triggers and how to avoid them."

- **Alicia, LPN**

Ah yes... triggers. It can be overwhelming living in a world where we can be set off at any time. For those with PTSD, most anything that reminds us of what happened right before or during a trauma is what can trigger a cascade of symptoms. It's not a very fun way to live and the stress often keeps us on edge and steals our hope of a better life. Triggers are usually tied to our senses – i.e. – we may see, feel, smell, touch, or taste something that brings on our symptoms. Some of the most common include:

Sounds: Hearing specific noises, music, or voices may bring back traumatic memories. For example, a car backfiring may remind a veteran of gunfire. My biggest sound trigger is a mother screaming in agony.

Smells: The sense of smell is closely tied to our memories. A house fire survivor may be triggered by the smoky smell from their neighbor's grill. The smell of burnt hair and gangrene get me every time.

Places: Understandably, returning to the scene of the trauma or visiting a place that reminds of it is often a big trigger. Any location though, like a deserted parking lot, might be enough to cause a reaction.

Touch/Sensation: Some feelings such as physical pain or touch are triggers. Assault survivors may have flashbacks as a result of being touched on a certain body part. I was choked by a psych patient once in the back of the ambulance and now am sensitive to anything being around my neck.

People/Things: Seeing a person or object that reminds you of the trauma may cause a PTSD response. We had a call where a kid hung himself in his room right next to a Metallica poster. Now every time I hear that band I think of him.

Thoughts/Emotions: Any new experience that makes you feel similar to the way you felt during a traumatic event (terrified, alone, helpless) could trigger symptoms. Feeling trapped or smothered in any way triggers me big time.

TV shows, news reports, and movies: In this day and age it's hard to find a television show or movie that doesn't depict violence. Seeing a similar trauma often sets off our symptoms.

Anniversaries: It's often hard to go through a date marked by trauma without remembering it. September 11th is a good example of this. Most all of us remember where we were that day…

How Can You Recognize Your Triggers?

One great way to recognize your trigger patterns is to keep a daily record or journal. Nobody knows your experience better than you do. Writing down how you feel and what you do each day can put you in the driver seat of your own experience. Seeing patterns in black and white can help us to realize where we need the most help. The notebook and tracking process doesn't have to be anything fancy. Just grab some paper and sit down for a few minutes every day to write it out. By keeping a record, you gain valuable insight into your own patterns, hot buttons and coping mechanisms. These insights can prove to be very valuable in combating your symptoms down the line. Documenting your triggers is one of the fastest and easiest ways to gain power over your experience by giving you the heads up on what sets you off. The Holistic PTSD Workbook that goes along with this book is a great option here too. It's got questions and prompts to help if you don't know where to start.

Let's be real - it is not fun walking around not knowing if or when you'll be set off. For many, the stress of trying not to be triggered can be one of the worst parts of their whole experience. Relax. It can change. Applying the tools in this book can help you regain the inner safety needed to heal beyond your triggers.

Now for a real-world practicum — Here are some quick tricks you can use to deal with symptoms and triggers: They only take a few minutes and can help interrupt the PTSD cascade in a pinch. As always, be your own advocate and only do what works for you.

Jump Up and Down. Don't laugh! This works. When you get caught up in your head, have anxiety, panic, depression, lethargy, or suicidal ideations, jumping up and down for five minutes (or until you feel better) on the ground or a rebounder trampoline can reset your energy and ground awareness back into your body.

Take a Cold Shower. Trust me, you'll learn to love this. Start with warm water and end your shower by turning the faucet to as cold as you can handle. Breathe deeply. Thirty seconds to two minutes in cold water can snap you out of your head and back into your body. Use this when anxiety/panic set in or if you have any urges to self-harm. Also recommended daily as an immune system booster.

Walk Barefoot Outside (On grass/dirt). Walk or lay down outside for ten to twenty minutes every day. It's called grounding or 'Earthing.' Check out the many in-depth studies and videos available online. There is a whole science behind it. The best part is that it's free and easy to do! Recommended daily as a preventative tool.

Breathing Technique: Inhale to the count of four and exhale to the count of six. Focus only on your breath. Repeat five to ten times. Focused breathing is one of the fastest ways to calm your mind and come back into the present moment. A shorter inhale and longer exhale mimics the way we breathe when we are asleep, and triggers the parasympathetic nervous system – which can help you get out of fight or flight response. Use any time you feel anxious, fatigued, depressed or panicked.

Emotional Freedom Technique (Tapping) is a combination of ancient Chinese acupressure and modern-day psychology that works to physically alter your brain, energy system, and body mechanics. The practice consists of tapping with your fingertips on specific meridian points. It can be done anywhere, anytime and often brings relief from difficult emotions quickly. Tapping can stop the fight or flight reaction by accessing the amygdala – the part of your brain that initiates your body's negative reaction to fear. It is simple and painless. You can apply it to yourself and can be done in a matter of minutes. You can find easy instructional videos on YouTube or check out Nick Ortner's site www.thetappingsolution.com.

Many people believe that PTSD is caused by a single traumatic event. While that can be true, I've learned through my research for this book that PTSD is often less about one singular instance than it may be about cumulative effect. Perhaps one instance becomes the proverbial straw that broke the camel's back — but years of long hours, irregular sleep cycles, and stressful situations really add up. Compound that with agency bureaucracy, toxic coworkers, passive-aggressive support staff, and power-tripping commanders and it's like working in a pressure cooker.

Real talk: there is often a deep pressure and apathy slithering through many departments and organizations. While some people put in thirty years and maintain their health and sanity – many do not. If we don't pay attention along the way, the systems and jobs that we love can drain us. While it's certainly not always the case, some might end up feeling disillusioned, like a cog in a wheel, stuck in a system that doesn't value them - or even outright discarded. It can be grim, the exhausting feeling that nothing will change no matter how many calls we run or tours we do. Again, not everyone feels this way – but dealing with the darkest elements of society day in and day out can definitely take a toll. If you are overworked, undervalued, sleep deprived, yelled at, scrutinized, feel stuck or are just biding time until retirement – your health and wellbeing can suffer. Sometimes we train for years to attain our dream position only to realize that it's not what we thought it would be...

It can all be a lot to deal with. Recognizing that you are not alone is an important part of the healing process. Whatever your experience, don't give up. You are a person of value who contributes a great deal to this world.

Again, we are **stronger together.**

■

"I'm a veteran mental health professional with PTSD. I served a combat tour in Afghanistan helping those who needed it, all the while wanting someone to ask me the same questions I was asking them. I was depressed, but pushed through, because that's just what you're expected to do. Knowing the pain that others felt made me too sad, and since coming home, things have only gotten worse. I feel numb, disconnected from everyone, even pets (I used to adore pets). I wear a mask to work, pretending to be happy because that's what I think I should be doing. I can't sleep without Ambien every single night. I feel like I should try harder to be normal. I don't know who I am. I miss the happy-go-lucky, carefree person that I used to be. I want that person back."

- Anonymous

The Standard Breakdown Process

You might be wondering, 'Are all first responders and military personnel destined to a life of PTSD?" The answer to that question is unequivocally NO. Being in our field can be incredibly rewarding. We see and do things that most people never even dream of, and often help people through their worst moments. Our careers can be long, healthy and deeply satisfying. We can raise our families under the umbrella of service work and pass good work ethic onto our kids. We can benefit from the camaraderie and form deep relationships with our brothers and sisters.

That said, if we don't take care of ourselves along the way we'll likely pay for it sooner or later. Sometimes the wear and tear on our bodies and minds creeps up slow and steady, other times it comes hard and fast. During my field time I noticed that many of my coworkers were great at helping others but didn't seem to take very good care of themselves. A few were committed to fitness early in their careers but over time most of them became distracted, lethargic, or focused on anyone but themselves. I listened to many of my friends complain over the years about aches and pains while eating nothing but fast food all day then going home and binge drinking at night. Several of my colleagues needed knee and shoulder replacement surgeries from on duty injuries, one had a heart attack at the station and another had a stroke.

As the years go by, the weight of a life of service can take its toll and it can be easy to let ourselves go. We are human and doing the best we can. I've certainly struggled with my own challenges. That said - if we remember to prioritize our own health and wellbeing throughout our careers, we can avoid breakdowns over time.

After all those countless hours in the ambulance chatting with different colleagues about life and death, likes, dislikes, worst calls, fears, dreams, relationships, family, and life on and off duty – I noticed a pattern: three distinct coping categories that most people fell into after being in service for a while. Some coworkers seemed to be functioning pretty well but still had elements of white knuckling life as workaholics, alcoholics or addicts. Others talked about being a bit more out of control: getting written up, being bankrupt, having toxic marriages or being estranged from their kids. Still others admitted to me that they were in *very* dark places and didn't want to do the job anymore but didn't know how to quit. Thousands of conversations spanning fifteen years helped me recognize three general categories first responders often experience: compensated (holding it together), decompensated (breakdown), and anarchy (blow up/end your life).

You might recognize the terms **compensated and decompensated** from the shock management protocol of a trauma patient. They seem to apply here too. These are not technical terms in this instance as much as a general spiral that we might take if we don't take care of ourselves during our careers. Again, not everyone is affected. Though not everyone ends up sliding down the rabbit hole, many do. Think about it: we are trained how to triage and take care of others, but we are often not adequately taught how to take care of ourselves in relation to the chaos and violence that we see. Remember, the stages are not absolute, nor does everyone move through them the same way. Some people take their entire career to get to decompensated state, while other newbies might go straight to anarchy after a series of bad calls or deployments. Some seem to breeze through their careers with little affect – again – it's all unique to the individual.

Here's a bit more information about each category. Can you relate? In which do you find yourself?

.

Compensated PTSD – Getting By

"I am cold as ice and come off rude to a lot of people. Defense mechanism. I just have zero tolerance for any crap now. I just want to live my life in peace. Some people just don't get that, so they get to see what happens when they trigger the PTSD. I am safer alone." **Jonathan, US Army Veteran**

The compensated category is where most of us live for years. This is when we can still function and handle business, show up for our families and crews, perform our job functions, and 'do what needs to be done' — even if we often don't feel good or know something is 'off.'

In the compensated stage it is common to:

- Ignore or suppress feelings
- Disconnect from or neglect our body
- Have a sense that something is wrong, but ignore it
- Push through – work harder
- Self-medicate with addictions
- Alcohol was the #1 reported coping mechanism while researching this book
- Working overtime #2
- Other extreme or addictive behaviors such as pills, gambling or affairs #3

Sam's Story

Sam was an EMT in my new-hire class in LA. Sitting directly behind me in orientation, I noticed that he couldn't ever seem to sit still or be quiet. Disheveled, he fidgeted constantly and talked incessantly to the people around him. His papers were everywhere, and he always had a stack of king-sized candy bars and a Big Gulp soda on his desk.

After three days of mostly trying to ignore his constant distractions, my classmates and I finally turned around to talk to him. Following a general nicety about where we were each being assigned for shift, Sam said matter-of-factly, 'I watched my dad kill my mom when I was ten.' Everyone was shocked into silence.

Not knowing how to respond at the time I eventually stuttered, 'Um… uh...did you… Did you ever get help for that?'

'Not really,' he said. 'I was put in foster care and they called 911 all the time for another boy who had seizures. That's how I decided that I wanted to be an EMT. Those firefighters who came to my house were always so nice to me. They made me feel like I mattered.' With that, our little group broke and we all went back to our desks with the disturbing knowledge that had been shared.

Bless his heart, Sam continued to be a fidgety mess during orientation but eventually graduated and was assigned the Inglewood division with me and two other recruits. For the next few years, I saw him in passing at the beginning of shift and in hospital bays when we were both dropping off our patients. He always looked the same: uniform shirt un-tucked, brown hair sticking out the top of his head, glasses tilted sideways on his face and his stethoscope hung loosely around his neck.

Many crews were mean, always hazing and playing pranks on him— but I always tried to be nice when I saw him. I felt bad, and in some way was glad that he told me about what he had been through as a kid. It helped me not be annoyed by him or his mannerisms. That wasn't the case for most, though, and Sam endured endless ridicule for years.

I was not surprised to hear that it eventually became too much for him. After one particularly bad shift, Sam had a nervous breakdown at work. A domestic violence turned murder-suicide call that he responded to pushed him over the edge. He broke down on scene and left EMS that day. Two years passed and I didn't hear anything more about him.

Then one Saturday morning I was at the grocery store when we randomly bumped into each other. I was astounded by what I saw. No longer a scraggly mess, Sam had lost sixty pounds and was well groomed. I barely recognized him, but he remembered me and struck up a conversation.

When I remarked on how good he looked, he told me that call had broken him in half and he had to leave the field to save his own life. He shared that he had immediately gotten himself into counseling and aggressive trauma therapy. He started meditating and took a significant interest in eastern medicine. It was a hard road, but he eventually came to terms with his childhood trauma and rebuilt his life. He had even enrolled in nursing school and had gotten engaged!

I was thrilled for him. Sam was someone who could have easily given up. He had the deck stacked against him from a young age and had been hazed throughout his EMS career, but despite all that had decided to take his life and fate back into his own hands. I was in awe of his tenacity. We hugged each other happily and parted ways. I still think of Sam with tremendous admiration for the hard work he put in to become the man he is today.

■

In some ways, Sam's breakpoint was a bit of grace because it forced him onto a better path. But there's no need to wait for your breaking point. I encourage you to do what you need to do to find help as soon as you notice you're compensating for PTSD symptoms.

Decompensated PTSD – Breakdown

"We get used to handling crazy situations by armoring our head and heart. We have to do it in order to cope. So we wall ourselves off – until our body and mind just can't handle anymore and everything starts to break down."

- Rick, Deputy Sheriff

To me, the decompensated stage is when we start to lose control and our lives go sideways. The coping mechanisms that may have worked for us no longer do and we find ourselves really struggling in order to maintain. Our bodies start to break down. We often get angry and impatient, and might have bouts of rage, apathy or depression. We stop doing things we used to love. Our thoughts, moods, and behavior become more and more unreliable. We drop the ball on important things in our lives and often experience self-loathing. We try like hell to keep it together to maintain our jobs and families, but we are often only partially successful.

In the Decompensated stage it is common to:

- Have erratic mood swings, anxiety or panic attacks
- Try even harder to keep everything afloat
- Engage in ever more risky and destructive behavior
- Lose control of our drinking or drug use
- Get written up or put on notice at work
- Lash out in anger and alienate family

Jeanette's Story

Jeanette grew up in a family where both her dad and grandfather had been battalion chiefs in the fire department and she decided early that she wanted to follow in their footsteps.

After completing junior academy at sixteen, she took part in an explorer program and spent her weekends doing ride-alongs. When she turned eighteen she earned her EMT license and put in several more years working before being hired to her dream job in the fire department.

The hazing began immediately for everyone in the new hire academy as the instructors attempted to 'wash out' new recruits. Prepared for that, Jeanette sucked it up and dealt with the yelling, pranks, and demeaning comments. She knew how to play the game and wasn't about to let anyone stand in the way of her goal.

She eventually graduated and began to shine in the department. For the next fifteen years Jeanette gave the fire service her all. Unfortunately, her passion wasn't fully reciprocated. Passed over by three times on the captain test, she saw the position go to lesser-qualified men. Being the only woman in her department was difficult. Her crew routinely excluded from off-duty activities, she was ignored and condescended on duty. They messed with her on scene by hiding equipment and yelling at her later for not being competent. Grinning and bearing it, she considered changing stations but resolved to just deal with it all on her own. The last thing she wanted was to tarnish her dad and grandfather's reputations by being the 'girl who whined.'

Years rolled by and the hazing took its toll. Jeanette eventually burned out. The calls that she had once loved running didn't do anything for her anymore, and she developed a negative attitude toward life.

Realizing that her childhood dream of rising through the ranks of the fire department would likely never happen, Jeanette started drinking every day. A beer or two initially, her habit quickly escalated to a bottle of vodka or more. Still resolved, she kept showing up for duty and going through the motions. She got by until one day she injured her back moving a 500lb man from his bed to the gurney. A fresh prescription of oxycodone followed.

What developed next was an unhealthy addiction to both alcohol and narcotics. No one knew the extent of her usage until the morning she didn't report for duty. A friend was sent to her house for a welfare check and found her unresponsive in bed. Jeanette had overdosed.

Fortunately, help arrived in time. She was revived and ultimately sent to rehab. Taking extended medical leave, she spent the next six months doing intensive therapy and support groups. Group therapy helped her realize how pride and her inability to ask for help spiraled her into resentment and addiction.

Slowly, she began taking responsibility for her choices and actions. Jeannette also realized that she used pills and alcohol to mask feelings of anger, inadequacy, and rejection.

Scared straight, she stepped up and took full responsibility for her life. Actively processing her pain, she engaged in trauma release exercises, regression therapy, and acupuncture. She cleaned up life, routinely went to AA meetings and developed a support system of people who held her accountable.

Ultimately, Jeannette returned to the fire service. Upon reentry, she decided not to go back to the status quo. Instead, she wanted to use her experience to contribute to the department in a different way. Jeannette launched PTSD support groups to help her coworkers with similar struggles. Instead of feeling ashamed, Jeanette turned her tragedy into triumph by using her story to help other people choose a better way.

Anarchy – Blow It All Up

"I was beyond pissed when I got forced out on medical retirement. After sacrificing everything for this country, I got cast aside like a dog when they were done with me. My wife left me too. She said her and the kids didn't even know me anymore. So I said 'fuck it.' What does it even matter? Next thing I know, I was arrested for attacking a police officer after washing down my painkillers with booze. I woke up in the clink with one hell of a hangover and a lot of regret."

- Jeff, Retired Air Force Staff Sergeant

Anarchy is what I call the stage where we have officially lost control and we blow up our lives a result. Those who never digress to this point are lucky. There's not a lot of fun to be had at this stage. For the unfortunate ones who do bottom out here, healing can seem dubious at best. Even if you find yourself all they way down and out, please do not give up hope. It will take some doing, but you can still climb out of the abyss. As long as you have a heartbeat and breath in your lungs – you still have a chance at a new life.

In the Anarchy stage it is common to:

- Develop significant and debilitating health issues
- Lose your job or rank
- Lose your friends and family
- Follow an addiction to the point of overdose, bankruptcy, or death
- Develop suicidal ideation or even follow through on suicide

Ted's Story

Jackie's husband Ted was with one of the first police officers on scene at an active school shooting. A first of its kind in the area (long before school shootings were commonplace), none of the crews on scene knew the extent of what they were walking into.

The stress level was extreme. Entering the main hallway in search of the shooter, they waded through pleading cries for help and bullet-riddled bodies of dead students littering the hallway. Ted later recalled experiencing an extreme sense of fear and helplessness that he had never felt before throughout his lengthy career. After a long and bloody standoff, the teenage shooter was eventually shot and killed. Several more hours of triage, patient transport, and

CSI set up ensued before Ted and his crew were finally debriefed and sent home.

After the incident, the department offered the standard critical incident stress management, which included further debriefing and counseling. But it was a drop in the bucket compared to what Ted actually needed. The day of the incident at school marked the beginning of his undoing.

He had coped relatively well with the stress of his job for years, but something about this call flipped a switch in his head and it was like all of his usual coping mechanisms stopped working. In the weeks and months following, Ted tried his best to downplay his experience. His buddies weren't saying anything, so he stayed quiet and tried his best to forget about it all and just get back to work.

But he couldn't. No matter what he did, he couldn't stop thinking about the dead kids in the hallway. Ted promptly went to the doctor and was prescribed four different medications for anxiety and insomnia. Those made him feel weird so instead he started drinking. Suffering greatly in silence, he continued working until the day he was dispatched to another shooting – where he promptly had a nervous breakdown. Ted was forced to retire out on medical disability.

Suddenly, Ted was home with his wife Jackie all the time. Not used to having him around so much, she didn't quite know how to handle it. He was a mess— unstable and volatile, flying between highs and lows with little in-between. He barked constantly and griped about everything from her cooking to the state of the country.

He quit showering, made messes everywhere, and wouldn't help with anything around the house. His mental state declined the more he drank. And he drank a lot.

Though frightened and a bit overwhelmed, Jackie did her best to keep the household running while supporting her husband. A police officer's wife for decades, she was used to his mood swings but had never experienced such severe outbursts before.

She put up with his behavior until one night she was jolted awake to find Ted poised above her with his hands clamping down around her throat. He appeared to be in some sort of delirium, muttering incoherently about killing the shooter.

Terrified, Jackie pushed him off and fled downstairs to call for help. Ted was put in an in-patient facility where he ultimately got sober and was given the intensive treatment he needed. Jackie visited him religiously. After four long months of intensive therapy, Ted was released.

Jackie was there waiting for him when he was discharged. With continued counseling and the support of friends and family, they were able to begin a new chapter of life together.

∎

Compensated → Decompensated → Anarchy

These generalized stages are an overview of the slippery slope and breakdown process that many of us face if we don't take care of ourselves consistently.

Please remember, we DO NOT have to go down this path. We can have long healthy, happy lives and careers if we are diligent about prioritizing ourselves over time.

Three Ways to Avoid the Spiral:

1. Be aware of red flags.
2. Take daily action to protect your health and wellbeing.
3. Be willing to ask for help.

You **can** change the outcome of your life by taking small steps every day to maintain balance in your body/mind and emotions. If you're thinking, 'It's *too late for me'* – please stop. As long as you are alive you can still change your life for the better. Now let's talk about how.

Introduction to Holistic Healing

"I work in healthcare and probably 40% of the oncology patients and their family members that I see can check off all the qualifying symptoms for PTSD. Any life-threatening situation can be processed in the brain and stored in a way that causes PTSD. The brain needs lots of help re-storing the memories in a better way...with less cortisol being brought up if a trigger happens. What has helped me the most is adding integral yoga and breathing practices in with other treatment. I believe for veterans, their families and civilians who experience life traumas that yoga and breathing practices, alongside cognitive treatment with a qualified therapist, will be part of a greater healing than what meds and therapy alone offer."

- Robyn, LPN

Chris' Story

Chris was an Army ranger who was raised by a meth-addicted mom in a tiny town in Oklahoma. Frequently left home alone, he watched over his three younger siblings and worked odd jobs whenever he could to help with money for groceries. Despite having little time for himself, Chris managed to graduate high school with honors. Dreaming of a better life, he enlisted in the army and shipped off to boot camp just two days after his graduation. He was nervous to leave but promised to call and send money back to help whenever he could. Halfway through his first year of training, Chris received the devastating news that his mom had overdosed, and his siblings were to go live with distant relatives. He wanted to help but also knew there was little he could do since they had already been sent away. Using his grief as fuel, Chris pushed himself to excel in the army. He wanted to prove to himself that he was better than his past. His goal was to eventually have enough money to help his brothers and sister get out of that small town and go to college. Through tremendous hard work, dedication, and sacrifice Chris eventually achieved his dream of becoming an Army ranger. Time clicked by and he served on multiple combat tours. On his final deployment, he was riding in a vehicle that rolled over an IED – killing ten people.

He lost his left leg, arm, and the vision in his left eye. After being held prisoner by local insurgents, he was eventually rescued by allies, stabilized, and transferred back to the states.

Upon being admitted into the VA system, Chris began having night terrors. Reliving the sights, sounds, and smells from the attack over and over, he stopped sleeping and developed chronic insomnia. Lying awake for hours at night, he also began blaming himself for his mom's death, thinking that if he hadn't enlisted in the Army his family would still be together. Tormented, his lack of sleep led to crippling anxiety, depression, and delusions. At his worst, he became paranoid of the nursing staff and often reacted aggressively toward them. Per standard protocol, Chris was given multiple heavy-duty medications to help manage his symptoms. The drug cocktails helped him sleep a bit, but they made him feel like a zombie. Physically and mentally exhausted, he developed severe body tremors, constipation, night sweats and a profound sense of anger and helplessness over his situation. After switching medications four times in six months with minimal relief, it all became too much. The grief, the guilt, his repeated visions… Chris hit his max. Just before change of staff at 0600 on a Thursday morning, the honored army ranger's body was found hanging in a single stall bathroom just down the hall from his room.

■

Chris's story is unfortunately all too common for our veterans. Wouldn't it be nice if a lifetime of trauma and pain could be fixed with a handful of pills? We know that's too simplistic, and yet that's often the focus of the standard treatment plan for PTSD. But if every instance of PTSD is different, with specific and unique triggers and symptoms, how can there be a "standard" treatment plan at all?

After a full career of following SOP, it can be incredibly demoralizing when the standard isn't working for you, when following the rules and following procedure just takes you in circles. But when someone says they can't help you, that doesn't mean you can't be helped. It means that one individual doesn't know *how* to help you. Don't give up! There are a lot more choices out there for you than you might realize. **Keep looking for help wherever you can and accept help wherever you find it.**

What is Holistic Healing Anyway?

Holistic healing works to bring all aspects of a person's body, mind, emotions and spiritual awareness back into balance. By addressing every level of the individual, the person is better able to heal the root cause of their ailment. While western medicine focuses mainly on symptom suppression and surgery, holistic healing actually encourages the person to dig down and tap into the origin of the trauma in order to finally release it from the body. Therefore, finally being able to potentially heal from it.

For the skeptics out there, I got you. There are many branches of holistic healing that pull heavily from anatomy, physiology, science and quantum physics. The more you know about the different types of healing modalities available, the more empowered you can become to find a treatment plan that addresses your individual and personalized needs.

Some types of holistic healing that are becoming popular in western culture:

EMDR

Meditation

Yoga

Energy Work

Reiki

Massage Therapy

Myofascial Release

Medical Intuition

Craniosacral Therapy

Acupuncture

Hypnotherapy

Naturopathy

Reflexology

Many, many more ...

In order to fully understand your options, it's good to know the three main types of medicine practiced globally. That way you can pull modalities specific to your needs from each branch to have a well-rounded and sustainable healing program tailored specifically to you. The three types of medicine practiced today are:

Modern Medicine - also known as allopathic or 'western' medicine focuses on individual body systems and the diagnosis and treatment of symptoms using interventions like drugs, radiation or surgery. This relatively new branch (only a few hundred years old) is amazing at trauma care, suppression of symptoms, and life-or-death emergencies. Chronic illness, pain management, and mental health—not so much.

If you are trying to manage your PTSD with only the tools of Modern Medicine, then that's likely all you will ever do: manage it. To truly heal and get beyond the pain, you will likely need to look further. And deeper.

Traditional/Eastern Medicine

Traditional medicine is thousands of years old and has withstood the test of time. The main focus Traditional/Eastern medicine is the integration of physical, mental and emotional health as well as spiritual wellbeing. Restoring health is seen as a process of bringing the individual's systems back into balance. It is gaining in popularity in the modern culture as preventative and corrective medicine. Every culture has their own legacy of traditional medicine, from the Ayurvedic physicians of India to the tribal shamans of North America. The most famous system, Traditional Chinese Medicine (TCM) is now practiced all over the world.

Energy/Holistic Medicine also seeks to bring body, mind, and spirit back into balance. Holistic healing has been around for millennia in different forms, but Energy Medicine as an organized medicine has only been around since the early 1980s. It is defined as any energetic interaction with a biological system that brings back balance to the organism. Dr. Oz famously said, "The next big frontier in medicine is Energy Medicine."

There are many types of energy medicine practiced today that utilize quantum physics and the subtle energy fields of the body for powerful healing. Since our bodies (and everything in our world) is made up of vibrational energy, working with a gifted healer who knows how to balance those energies can bring powerful transformation from the inside out. I work with clients all over the world in my private energy healing practice and have been amazing time and again by the incredible transformation they can experience with Energy Medicine.

•

Each of these branches of medicine has their pros and cons. To me, no one type of medicine is better than another because they all offer such different approaches to healing and wellness. Some of the most powerful recoveries I've ever witnessed in clients and friends programs happen when the person takes bits from all three branches and formulates a plan that suits their individual needs. Our western culture isn't often taught much about different options, and that's why I've written this book. I'm happy to share all I know with you so you can feel more informed and empowered in your own health and life.

True healing is messy business.

Many people avoid taking steps to finally heal themselves because the process often doesn't feel very good. True healing – like, to-your-core healing – isn't as much blissful as it is gritty.

I'm not trying to scare you off as much as speak truth and prep you for the journey. In addition to not being educated on options, our culture isn't often taught how to be still and navigate the wealth of trauma lodged in our bodies and minds. Instead, we are rewarded for relentless striving and encouraged to medicate away any pesky symptoms that don't feel good…

I am certainly not anti-western medicine and believe that there is definitely a time and place for appropriate medication and surgery. That said, much of our system is set up to have medication as the go-to protocol. And those med don't work, the providers often want to medicate even more! It's kind of crazy when we stop and think about it. Fortunately, more and more people are growing tired of the hamster wheel and are looking for other, more natural ways to help themselves feel better.

Again, everyone is unique and responds differently to different programs. I encourage you to open your mind to the vast world of possibilities out there. By expanding our scope and pulling from all available western and alternative modalities, we can tailor custom plans for maximum success.

In the next few chapters, I will introduce different modalities from Traditional and Energy Medicine to help with your specific issues.

Healing From PTSD

"I survived a suicide attempt this summer. Before that I had been pretty stable for about ten years. So I'm going to tell you what I'm doing now. Talk therapy, every other week. I don't isolate. I attend church, Sunday school, Guitars for Vets... I don't watch violence and I take my medicine. Exercise. I call my Mom a lot. I'm not perfect. But I go with what I know."

- Judith – Army Private

A solid and basic foundational understanding and routine is paramount in the healing process. Just like most 911 calls, the vast majority of treatment required is basic. The same can be said for your PTSD integration. More aggressive and advanced tools will be provided, but having a solid routine set in your daily self-care is key to a lasting positive impact.

Overcoming PTSD is possible. What it requires from you is 100% accountability for your life and situation. I get that you've been to hell and back, but the question now is: What are *you* willing to do about it? Your mindset here is critical. Making new, small choices and actions every day can change your circumstances. Please also remember that no one can do it for you. The outcome of your life and your healing are your own responsibility. This can be a bitter pill to swallow after everything that you've been through, but willingness to take ownership of every aspect of your life puts the power back in your hands. It's tempting and easy to slide into victim mentality, but in order to heal we must reclaim our power.

Start simply. Even twenty minutes a day of a new choice or behavior can change the direction of your life. Once you feel better, you will have more energy available to tackle the bigger challenges.

Additionally, this is a marathon, not a sprint. The tools in this book are the foundation. You don't have to do all of them, just choose one or two and start there. They can be used to cope with existing PTSD, as well as to prevent further issues from developing.

I highly recommend that you have a regular daily self-care routine established, a support system of friends and family in place, and have a healer or therapist on hand as you embark upon your healing journey. And please, don't forget to laugh a little along the way. You've been through so much darkness and chaos that letting yourself be a bit less serious from time to time can work wonders in your life. It's alright to let down a little… promise.

Again, I'm not a doctor or shrink so I can't diagnose you or tell you any one definitive way to heal from your PTSD. What I am is a first responder who has done it, so I figured I'd just tell you what I did and let you go from there. Remember, everyone is different. What works for you might not for someone else, and that's okay. Once you understand different healing options, you can take it one step at a time to develop a protocol that works specifically for you.

It took me years of diligent effort to heal myself. The reason it took so long was because I'm stubborn and wouldn't let anyone tell me what to do so I was out there trying everything I could find. ☺ Some things really helped. Others did not. Some things were legit, others proved to be nonsense. But I kept at it. I tried everything that sounded interesting until eventually I realized that I had rounded the corner from 'trying to heal' to 'being healed.' With little fanfare at all, I had arrived. I woke up feeling great. My anger and flashbacks disappeared, I softened and let people close to me, my body and nervous system recovered, I no longer hated humanity, and most excitingly, I found a new purpose and direction for my life. I'm certainly not perfect, but I can sure tell you that the journey back into my power has been well worth it. You can do it too. I really do believe that. I believe in you. Whether you think yourself to be too far gone - or perhaps that you don't need any help at all! - the rest of this book contains powerful tools that come help you change your life beginning right now.

Many say it cannot be done—but I am living proof that healing from PTSD is possible.

To heal ourselves we must tackle each of these five very important areas:

1) Restore biochemistry of the brain

Stress physically changes the brain. To overcome PTSD, we have to restore our brain chemistry so that we can rest and process through the events and triggers.

2) Release trauma from the body

Trauma is stored in the body. Just talking about it isn't enough. We need to physically move it out of our cells to heal.

3) Process difficult emotions

You have to feel it to heal it. This is often people's least favorite – but it is essential to overcoming PTSD.

4) Reclaim physical health

Rebuilding physical health and vitality goes hand in hand with healing.

5) Establish a new identity beyond the trauma

Establishing a new, healthy identity beyond what happened to you and what rank you held is a pivotal point for life beyond PTSD.

***

If you take nothing else away from this book, please remember these five key areas! The upcoming chapters explain each area in detail and give you recommended holistic modalities to try. You don't have to do them in any particular order, though establishing a new identity beyond the trauma often comes last after working through the other items.

Believe in yourself! You are worth fighting for! It's your turn to feel good... Are you ready?

HOLISTIC PTSD RECOVERY

Find what works for you.

Restore Biochemistry of the Brain

Brainspotting / EMDR
Binaural Audio
Biofeedback
Hypnotherapy
Breathing Techniques

Release Trauma from the Body

Craniosacral Therapy
Trauma Release Exercises (TRE)
Float Tanks
Myofascial Release
Reiki

Process Difficult Emotions

Somatic Trauma Therapy
Meditation
Acupuncture
Journaling
Rage Release Exercises

Reclaim Physical Health

Nutrition
Hydration
Sleep/ Exercise
Infrared Sauna

Establish a New Identity

Neurolinguistic Programming (NLP)
Intuitive Coaching
Visualization Techniques
Try Something New
Do Something You Think You Can't

5 Ways to Restore Biochemistry of the Brain

"Bad things happen to good people every day. It's how we react to the bad stuff and frame it in our mind that ultimately heals or destroys us."

- Jacob, NYPD

Hang with me for just a bit of anatomy; I'll try to make it painless and it will play a role in helping you understand your symptoms. The prefrontal cortex is located in the frontal lobe just behind your forehead. The PFC is designed to regulate attention and awareness, helps with decision-making and discernment, regulates emotions, and inhibits dysfunctional reactions. When you take a practical exam, meet with your boss, or talk your way out of a speeding ticket, that's your PFC in action. But when you see something out of the corner of your eye barreling down on you, you have less than a second to determine if this is the guy who stole your girlfriend (fight!) or a charging bear (flight!). There isn't time to engage the prefrontal cortex, so instead the decision is sent to the amygdala. If you've ever found yourself acting before your awareness caught up, before you knew why you were acting, that was the amygdala taking the wheel. After the prefrontal cortex yields to the amygdala, its function will be reduced for a time. This is called inhibition or down-regulation. For a little while, higher reasoning will be more difficult, which can make it hard to remember that starting a bar fight will get you into trouble, or that there's a fence between you and that bear. When you're under the control of the amygdala, decisions get made fast, but they're not necessarily the best decisions.

When overly activated, the body stays in perpetual fight-or-flight. Hyper-stimulation of the nervous system then makes it virtually impossible to switch control back to the PFC. When the prefrontal cortex stays inhibited, erratic mood swings, unpredictable thoughts, and diminished control over your actions could result. These can create imbalances in your body as well as personality changes. These changes may be permanent unless significant action is taken by you to reclaim your life and power.

This is key because getting out of sympathetic response and into a more restful state of mind is necessary for beginning the healing process. The downshifting of the PFC is useful for functioning under stress, running toward danger, and other common factors necessary for the job, but the prefrontal cortex cannot shift between 'on' and 'off' very easily. You might live a double life between work and home, but your PFC does not. Many of the symptoms of PTSD are due to a down-regulated PFC. The goal is not to turn it all the way back up as that would impede our ability to do our jobs. That said, by understanding what is actually happening in your brain you can empower your healing process.

In addition to fight-or-flight, the amygdala also plays a role in memory formation. This is why our clearest memories are times of great stress and emotionally charged experiences. You probably have a memory that is still crystal clear, like it happened yesterday. Every detail is still fresh, and it is possible to fall back into that memory like a "flashback." I shared one of mine at the start of this book. Like a groove in a record, the brain replays the trauma over and over.

Here is the down and dirty about your brain:

1)   When under chronic stress, the biochemistry of the brain changes.

2)   The amygdala (fight or flight response center) gets stuck 'on', and prefrontal cortex (higher reasoning center) is inhibited.

3)   Synaptic pathways in the brain become entrenched with the pattern of the trauma, as the memory plays over and over.

4)   These changes make it difficult to 'just get over it' because the brain is physically and chemically different.

5)   The brain is plastic, meaning capable of change. You don't have to be stuck this way.

The rest of this chapter shows you how. **Here are 5 powerful ways you can help reset your brain chemistry:**

Brainspotting/EMDR

"I have been undergoing EMDR therapy for almost a year and it is tough and takes time. But it works and is well worth it. If you're a Veteran you know the term - Embrace The Suck"

Dan, US Army Combat Medic

EMDR (Eye Movement Desensitization and Reprocessing) is a psychotherapy practice that has really surged in popularity for helping clients with PTSD. EMDR helps people heal from the symptoms and emotional distress from trauma. Studies have shown that a few sessions of EMDR therapy can provide benefits that once took years of psychotherapy to attain. During EMDR, the client thinks about emotionally disturbing material in brief sequential doses while simultaneously being guided to focus on external stimuli. The therapist often directs lateral eye movements and uses hand-tapping and audio stimulation to help the person stay present as they process traumatic experiences. Using their extensive training and detailed protocols, clinicians help clients activate their own natural healing processes in a single session or a series. EMDR is safe, affordable, and has become a primary modality used to help people with PTSD. For more information, visit www.emdr.com.

Binaural Audio

'The immediate psychological effects on memory, attention, stress, pain, headaches and migraines were shown to benefit from even a single session.'
-*Excerpt from* <u>*A Comprehensive Review of the Psychological Effects of Brainwave Entrainment*</u>
Tina L Huang, PhD, and Christine Charyton, PhD

Binaural beats is a type of music or beat pattern that can help reset your brain by taking you into a meditative state. Binaural beats introduce stimulus to both hemispheres of the brain simultaneously. The brain goes from beta (conscious awareness) into theta (deep sleep/meditative state). Binaural audio is quick, easy, and potent. All you need to do is put on your headphones, sit or lie in a comfortable position, relax and let the sound heal you. This practice may be best utilized at night as you are preparing for sleep. My favorite binaural beats are Solfeggio Frequencies. You can find them for free on YouTube. Just type in Solfeggio PTSD (for anxiety, insomnia, depression etc.) and a list of videos will appear. Pick the one you like, put in your ear buds, and relax for 20-30 minutes – or until your triggers subside. Another good resource is www.hemi-sync.com, the official website for binaural beats music.

Biofeedback

> "I was having really bad nightmares and flashbacks when I came home from overseas. I couldn't sleep, was drinking a lot and was moody as hell. My girlfriend got sick of it and made try biofeedback. I thought it was hocus pocus at first, but I gotta say — it really helped me out."
>
> **Brent – Naval Officer**

Biofeedback is a mind-body technique that involves using visual or auditory feedback to gain control over involuntary bodily functions. This may include gaining voluntary control over such things as heart rate, muscle tension, blood flow, pain perception and blood pressure. Biofeedback can help teach awareness, ways to relax, and how to manage anxiety. It also helps reduce and control stress response. During a biofeedback session, electrodes are attached to your skin. Finger sensors can also be used. These electrodes/sensors send signals to a monitor, which displays a sound, flash of light, or image that represents your heart and breathing rate, blood pressure, skin temperature, sweating, or muscle activity. Your session will be dependent on what you need. For more information visit www.aapb.org.

Hypnotherapy

"After retiring from 30 years in the military, I had a hard time adjusting to civilian life. I missed the structure, my friends, and feeling like I had a purpose. I was like a fish out of water and just didn't seem to fit in to the regular world. Things got real bad for me for a while. An acupuncturist I was going to for chronic pain recommended hypnotherapy. I was skeptical at first, thinking I'm not interested in being brainwashed. She pointed out that I really didn't have much to lose since I was already struggling so much. I took a chance and am so glad I did it! Not only was it not weird like I expected, but it also relaxed and helped me sleep. The best part is that my mind changed. Like, all the years of thinking about the bad shit faded away. It's like I have a new brain now and I even have a bit of hope about my future. Who would have known that hypnotherapy could be so helpful?" **Ken – Marine Sergeant**

Hypnotherapy is guided hypnosis that is used to facilitate positive change by reframing thoughts, reactions, and addiction patterns. Regression Therapy is guided hypnosis designed to regress you back to a specific traumatic event in order to work through it, process, and heal. Although there are different techniques, clinical hypnotherapy is generally performed in a calm, therapeutic environment. The therapist will guide you into a relaxed, focused state and ask you to think about experiences and situations in positive ways that can help you change the way you think and behave. Unlike some dramatic portrayals of hypnosis in movies, books, or on stage, you will not be unconscious, asleep, or in any way out of control of yourself. To find a reputable hypnotherapist, you can visit www.natboard.com.

Breathing Techniques

"I didn't realize until my wife pointed out that I hold my breath a lot. She was watching me work on an engine and noticed. She asked me why I do that and I didn't really know. It wasn't until I was back on duty running a fatal car accident that I realized I was holding my breath again — this time because of the chaos. I figured out that's probably why I do it — stress. Since then, I've intentionally tried to breathe better. My headaches went away and I feel better overall." **Mark – Engineer**

Most of us don't breathe well. I know that sounds strange, but we are often so stuck in fight or flight that we take in little sips of air instead of filling our lungs and body with deep breaths. One of the fastest and most effective ways to change and calm your mind is by taking full, deep intentional breaths multiple times a day. Doing so oxygenates the brain and engages the parasympathetic nervous system, which calms you down. Once that happens, you can finally begin to process your thoughts and feelings to help your brain recover.

Just start with conscious breathing twice a day. Inhale to the count of four, then exhale to the count of four – repeat that in cycles of ten twice a day. It's free, relatively easy and can be done wherever you are. Just start by sitting upright, relaxing your neck and shoulders then inhaling so deeply that your belly expands. Exhale normally and relax. Repeat. Your body might feel tight and it may be challenging at first but the tension is where the trauma is stuck. The more energy and breath you send there, the more the frozen pain can soften and release. Try that for a week and see what comes up. You might be surprised just how powerful your breath can be.

5 Ways to Release Trauma from the Body

'My observations of scores of traumatized people has led me to conclude that post-traumatic symptoms are, fundamentally, incomplete physiological responses suspended in fear. Reactions to life-threatening situations remain symptomatic until they are completed. Post-traumatic stress is one example. These symptoms will not go away until the responses are discharged and competed. Energy held in immobility can be transformed with quietness, safety, and the feeling of protection.'

- From *Waking the Tiger* by Peter A. Levine

You know that feeling when the pressure is so high that everything goes silent? Things around you are literally blowing up or falling apart but to you it all is moving in slow motion? That is the moment when the psyche can't take anymore and often disassociates to protect itself.

We can still function and do what we need to do, but after the event subsides there is often a weird hollow feeling that sets in. That's likely because our body is trying to adjust to such a high level of intensity. All the stress and pressure gets pushed out of the way for a moment so that we can do our job, but that energy needs to be discharged soon after or it will get stuck in the nervous system.

In the wild, animals have a built-in release where they literally shake off trauma. When a deer narrowly escapes becoming a bobcat's dinner, it shakes itself to release the stress of the chase once it is safe. Animals instinctively know how to let go of the stress they just endured.

Humans are the only mammals that don't release trauma soon after the event occurred. Instead, we 'soldier on' as though nothing happened, stuffing all of the stress down into our bodies. Over time, that frozen pain creates physical symptoms: muscle tension, headaches, joint issues, ulcers, insomnia, anxiety, depression and flashbacks all indicate stress stuck in the body.

To heal, we must physically release the trapped tension from our cells.

Here are five great ways to do that:

Craniosacral Therapy

"Craniosacral therapy really helps my back and neck pain from years of stress and lifting heavy patients."

– Kim, EMT

CranioSacral Therapy (CST) is a gentle, hands-on approach that releases tensions deep in the body to relieve pain and dysfunction and improve whole-body health and performance. It was pioneered and developed by osteopathic physician John E. Upledger. Using a soft touch, practitioners release restrictions in the soft tissues that surround the central nervous system. CST is increasingly used as a preventive health measure for its ability to bolster resistance to disease, and it's effective for a wide range of medical problems associated *with* pain and dysfunction. By normalizing the environment around the brain and spinal cord and enhancing the body's ability to self-correct, CranioSacral Therapy is able to potentially alleviate a wide variety of dysfunctions, from chronic pain and sports injuries to stroke and neurological impairment. For more information visit www.upledger.com.

Tension and Trauma Release Exercises (TRE*)

"TRE is awesome. I started doing it because my shoulders hurt and I clenched my jaw all the time. It's crazy how much my muscles shake when I do it and how relaxed I feel afterward. I feel better – not as wound up."

- Jon, Corrections Officer

Dr. David Berceli is the creator of a system called Tension and Trauma Release Exercises (TRE), which are physical movements that trigger nervous system support and trauma release from the body. There are many ways to facilitate these releases. These simple yet potent exercises initiate shaking or vibrating that soothe muscle and organ tension, calm the nervous system, and invite the body back into balance. The exercises are relatively simple (wall squat, bridge pose, etc.) and can be done anywhere, anytime, and only take a matter of minutes to complete. As you go through the series, painless body tremors indicate that the process is working. Many people report feeling calm and lighter after undergoing the trauma release exercises. Once learned, this tool can be used independently as needed to manage and overcome symptoms of PTSD. For more information visit TraumaPrevention.com.

Float Tanks

"I don't like confined spaces so the idea of floating in a dark tank freaked me out at first, but then they told me I can keep the lights on and music playing if I want. So I tried it. My brain usually goes a million miles an hour but after the first few minutes I was actually able to relax a bit. It was nice — kinda like taking a break from my life for a while."

- Kevin, SFPD

Floatation, also known as sensory deprivation, is the act of relaxing in a floatation tank filled with warm water mixed with Epsom salt. The extreme buoyancy that individuals experience when floating is essentially like experiencing anti-gravity, which assists in drifting into a meditative state that rejuvenates your mind and body. This helps to calm your nervous system and enhances your body's natural ability to heal. The deep relaxation state that you enter when floating helps to reduce stress by lowering cortisol levels. Blood flow is stimulated and endorphins are released. Studies have shown that floatation therapy can even help with depression. The endorphins released during a float last beyond the float session itself. To find a float spa near you, check online.

Myofacial Release

"Myofacial release is the reason I can walk upright after a debilitating back injury on the job."

- Mike, Flight Medic

Myofacial release can be painful but is so worth it! It is a type of treatment treating skeletal muscle immobility and pain by relaxing contracted muscles, improving blood, oxygen, and lymphatic circulation, and stimulating the stretch reflex in muscles. By using firm pressure on specific areas of the body, a skilled practitioner can help release tightness in the connective tissues (fascia) to diminish pain, increase range of motion and relieve tightness that causes muscle constriction. Clients often experience significant relief from chronic symptoms after treatment. To find a myofacial release practitioner near you, go to www.myofascialrelease.com or check with your local massage therapist/sports therapist.

Reiki

"I was skeptical of reiki at first. Like, really? What kind of crap is this? But I was at the end of my rope with insomnia and flashbacks so I decided to give it a go. It's hard to describe what it feels like… relaxing I guess. All I know is that I slept a solid eight hours after my first session and have been going back ever since."

– Josh, Navy Seal

Reiki is rapidly becoming known in Western culture as a primary branch of energy healing. It is a very gentle and specific form in which hands are placed just off the body or lightly touching the body, as in "laying on of hands." Dr Mikao Usui introduced reiki in 1922. In a session, the client relaxes quietly as the practitioner infuses 'universal life energy' to the client. People often become deeply relaxed, fall asleep or have 'aha moments' that facilitate deeper insight and understanding about their pain. The benefits of reiki are vast and can be used to treat a wide array of symptoms from chronic pain to depression and anxiety. For more information or to find a reiki near you, visit www.iarp.org.

5 Ways to Process Difficult Emotions

"Four tours in Iraq and Afghanistan changed me. I became angry and closed off. I hated what I had seen and done. I thought not talking about it would make it go away, but it only made it worse. After drinking myself into oblivion for almost a year, I hit bottom. When my wife gave me an ultimatum, I finally went to get help. I thought talking about feelings was for pussies – but actually it was a key in me getting better. I still hate talking about the things I saw but now I know that keeping it locked up inside me would have killed me."
- **Brian, Army Ranger**

Dealing with difficult feelings is often one of the most challenging things for first responders and military personnel to do. Trained to perform under pressure, we set our personal feelings aside repeatedly in order to be of service. In our culture, emotional pain equals weakness and weakness equals death. We are typically reluctant if not blatantly unwilling to show vulnerability because that would threaten our identity in the field.

What we don't realize is that difficult feelings are a normal part of the human experience and keeping them locked away only causes complications down the line. When we don't acknowledge our emotions, we become apathetic, distant, cold, reactive and disconnected. We shut down, wall off and soldier on. We ignore, repress, self-medicate, and push through until something snaps—whether it be a physical or mental breakdown, a relationship ending, or some other event that forces us to finally address the deep well of pain within us.

When dealing with emotion it is important to note that there is no right or wrong way to do it. Some of us are so disconnected that we can't feel anything beyond a general apathy. Others are chronically depressed or fly off the handle at the smallest infraction. Just start where you are. It takes courage to face your emotions, especially when you've been conditioned to ignore them. Seeking the help of a trained professional can help you navigate these foreign waters and ease into the transition of a life beyond pain.

Here are five great ways to deal with your difficult feelings:

Somatic Trauma Therapy

"Somatic trauma therapy literally saved my life. I couldn't feel anything for years, like zero emotion. I went to some really dark places in my head and just wanted to die. Somatic trauma therapy helped me dig myself out of that hole and back into the world. I still struggle, but it's nothing like it used to be. I actually feel alive for the first time in a long time."

- Chris, Arson Investigator

Why is it that we can spend years in therapy and never really change? If all we do is talk, we might feel better in the moment, but typically go right back to the way it was after the session.

Somatic trauma therapy goes far beyond just talk therapy. This type of therapy focuses on gently drawing the trauma up out of the mind and body then releasing it from the body and nervous system through various pressure points, movements and releases. This is cutting-edge technique is leading the way in trauma recovery worldwide and is proving to be very effective in helping people with advanced cases of PTSD. I *highly recommend* this type of therapy in your recovery process. Peter Levine is the leading researcher and practitioner in this field. For more information, check out his work at www.traumahealing.org.

Meditation

"I used to think meditation was for sissies – until I tried it. Sitting still is hard because there's nowhere for me to run or hide when all my demons come out swinging. Meditation taught me that the real war is in my own mind and by taming it I can overcome even the worst experiences from my past."

- Rob, Firefighter

Meditation is a technique of calming the mind and connecting to your own experience. Meditation has been recorded as far back as 1500 BCE and is gaining popularity in current Western culture as a way to deal with external stress. Many people I interviewed for this book said they had tried meditation but couldn't get their mind to shut up, so they quit. Others said they were scared to be alone with themselves, so they wouldn't do it. I get it. The thought of facing our stuff can be overwhelming.

When I started meditating, I was so jumpy that I couldn't sit still so I started by listening to guided meditations. Listening to a soothing voice calmed me down. Positive change happened quickly. Within a week I became less tense, snappy, and even started to feel good. Eventually I felt confident enough to try more advanced techniques. Now, **I advocate meditation as one of the most powerful healing tools available.** The good news is that meditation is dose dependent. **Even a few minutes two or three times a week can begin the process of healing**. Another positive is that there are many kinds of meditation to choose from. Not every kind works for every person so it's good that there are options.

Research types of meditation and then find a local yoga studio or meditation center that offers what you want. YouTube has many great meditation videos available if you want to meditate at home. Use discernment and pick meditations from reputable companies. Chopra Center Meditations and Gaiam Meditations are very good, and I even created a guided meditation series specific for PTSD for first responders that you can find on my website.

Acupuncture

"Five treatments of acupuncture got me off my meds and fixed the back pain that the doctors said I'd have to have surgery for."

- Jesse, Coast Guard

Acupuncture has become quite common for treating PTSD. Acupuncture is a system of integrative medicine that involves sticking the skin or tissues with needles to influence the meridian and energy flow throughout the body. Acupuncture has withstood the test of time and is now widely accepted and available throughout the west. During a typical treatment, the practitioner introduces long acupuncture needles into the skin in specific areas of the body. The procedure is relatively painless. One set, the client will typically rest quietly for a period of time as the needles reset their meridian flow and energy systems. Sometimes the acupuncturist will introduce a soothing heat lamp, or he/she may tap, twist, or add more needles during the treatment. Significant relief can be found after a single session, though a series may be necessary depending on severity of the case. Acupuncture can now be found as an adjunct therapy in many hospitals. Fortunately, insurance is starting to cover sessions as well. Check online to find a good acupuncturist near you.

Journaling

"Writing shit down clears my head."

- Jeff, Bomb Squad

I love this one because you don't need any outside help to do it. Journaling is the process of writing down your internal thoughts and experience on paper. It doesn't have to be anything fancy. The whole point is to draw the chaos out of your mind and body by writing it down in a notebook or on a piece of paper. You can journal about anything: worries, anxieties, addictions, pain, daily stress… whatever. The process often helps us feel better because we can offload some of the pressure we face every day. Journaling regularly can help decrease anxiety and stress, increase emotional intelligence, identify triggers, addiction patterns, hopes and dreams.

Rage Release Exercises

"I've been angry all my life. Bar fights and back alley brawls used to get my aggression out, but I started getting in trouble so I stopped. Eventually my anger grew to blind rage. It wasn't until after my third divorce did I realize I had a problem. I found a good therapist and she recommended I release my anger responsibly. Now I punch heavy bags and spar at the gym. Crazy how much calmer it makes me when I do it often enough."

- Micah, SWAT

This is one that you can do on your own. Rage release exercises are exactly what they sound like: intentionally tapping into and releasing anger from the body. Too much anger festers and can cause all kinds of issues— from insomnia to impulse control problems to depression to physical pain. When we start to move our anger out, we can access the underlying emotions and fatigue within the body.

A few great rage release exercises are:

- Taking a baseball bat to a mattress
- Punching a heavy bag
- Smashing glass
- Shooting guns
- Rolling down the car windows while driving and yelling

These all feel amazing and can really free up some space for healing. That said, **be responsible**! Do not engage these behaviors around your family, kids, or bystanders! Moving rage out can be an explosive experience that can be very jarring to people around us. Please take responsibility and proceed with these exercises accordingly.

5 Ways to Restore Physical Health

"I was so angry when I retired out on disability. All my skills and training… for what? Things got really bad in my head for a while and I seriously considered killing myself. As a last resort my girlfriend signed me up for trauma therapy and helped me change my diet. I quit drinking, started eating better and lifting weights again. It took a while, but the nightmares finally stopped. I thought it was bullshit at first, but then it really started to help. After six months, I finally feel better and am starting to see a life beyond the Navy."
- Justin, Retired Navy SEAL

I know, I know—you've heard this a million times: your body is your temple. That's because it's true. To heal from PTSD, we must take care of our physical bodies. What we eat and drink and how we sleep literally affects our entire life. Physical health is the foundation for wellness. We cannot have one without the other. Eating well and attaining GI health have been shown to be among the fastest and most accessible ways to combat stress, disease, and PTSD symptoms.

Now, I am a realist and know that most first responders and military personnel are fueled by caffeine, sugar and alcohol. I also know that many of you won't give those up without a fight. That's fine, for now. This is not about taking away coping mechanisms as much as it is about establishing a solid foundation on which to build a healthy lifestyle. As far as diet, shift work can be brutal. Back when I ran twenty+ 911 calls in 24 hours, we'd be lucky to eat one meal and it was usually Taco Bell or whatever we could grab. Do your best. Just know that restoring your physical health is key in your healing process.

Here are five great ways to restore your physical health:

Nutrition

"A healthy outside starts from the inside."

Robert Urich

A diet consisting of high quality, organic, non-GMO food is optimal but not always realistic for field workers or those on deployment. Again, just do your best. I offer that you find some relatively healthy snacks (non-nitrate jerky, almonds, cashews, string cheese, fresh fruit, organic veggies, etc.) and keep them with you to eat between calls. When on base or deployment, you might consider requesting a 'care package' from friends or family with such ingredients so that you have access to food outside MRE's or what is available at the commissary. When home, maybe try following the 80/20 rule. Eat 'clean' by limiting sugar/refined starch/processed food 80 percent of the time, and let yourself indulge the other 20 percent. I've always found that eating well most of the time while letting myself 'live a little' helps me stay on track. Everyone's body is different. Use your best judgment and understand that quality nutrition and GI health are among the most efficient ways to increase your overall health and balance your body systems. Check out www.internalwisdom.com for custom holistic nutrition and wellness programs.

Hydration

"Now that's what I call high-quality H20."

- Bobby Boucher, *The Waterboy*

Here's another one that we hear about all the time—with good reason! Most people need six to eight 8oz glasses of water a day to stay properly hydrated. The amount varies per person, however, depending on body size, stress levels, and exercise habits. One easy rule of thumb is to **drink one glass of water for every cup of coffee or beer you have each day**. That little addition can go a long way. If staying hydrated is hard for you, here are some tips that can help:

When you're feeling hungry, drink water. Thirst is often confused with hunger. True hunger will not be satisfied by drinking water.

Drink on a schedule. Drink water when you wake up, at breakfast, lunch, and dinner, and when you go to bed. Or, drink a small glass of water at the beginning of each hour.

Keep a bottle of water with you during the day. To reduce your costs, carry a reusable water bottle.

If you don't like the taste of plain water, try adding a slice of lemon or drops of bitters, or drink sparkling water for that extra punch.

Sleep

"I want to sleep but my brain won't stop talking to itself."

– Michael, Miami PD

Ah yes, the elusive 'S' word.

It may come as no surprise that sleep ranks among the very top factors required for health and vitality. Studies show that getting seven to eight hours of sleep a night is vital to brain function, body system restoration, and immune health.

Lack of sleep is known to be a primary contributing factor for many chronic health conditions including anxiety and depression. Unfortunately, shift work can really mess up the circadian rhythms of the body. Being deployed, on patrol, at the prison, or up running calls all night throws off the natural sleep cycle and often makes it hard to get the deep rest we need.

Standard modern medical treatment for insomnia is to prescribe medication. Pills may help for the short-term, but dependency, addiction, and ugly side affects are commonly reported. If you take meds to sleep and they genuinely help you, great! If you have been on them for a while and want off, or are looking for more natural way, here are a few well-known supplements that you can try:

Melatonin - Hormone that regulates the sleep-wake cycle by telling the body that it is almost time for bed. It is available in capsules and liquid form at most health food stores and online. To avoid feeling sleepy the next day, be mindful of dose and ingestion time.

CBD - Cannabidiol that is a non-psychoactive component of hemp and cannabis. Recorded as a sleep agent as far back as 1200 A.D. in Chinese medical text and has been clinically proven to reduce anxiety and pain. Grey area in terms of legality and licensure! Be aware of your agency policy and make informed choices. Available online and at legal dispensaries.

Valerian Root – Plant with medicinal properties that have been extracted from the root and used by humans as a sleep aid since the days of ancient Greece and Rome. Available in teas, capsules, and liquid form– over the counter at most health food stores and online.

Exercise

"It hurts now but one day it will be your warm-up."

– Jack, Fire Captain

Movement is critical to wellbeing! Even 20 minutes a day can help prevent injury, reduce stress, boost endorphins, and promote better sleep – all of which have been shown to decrease the effects of PTSD. Sitting in an ambulance or on base for weeks, months, or years can be terrible for your body.

Plainly stated: use it or lose it. If you don't move, your body will eventually break down. Muscles and joints tighten, pull, and pop out of alignment and you might end up facing an otherwise preventable shoulder or back surgery. How many guys do you know retired out due to preventable injury? Probably a lot.

When it comes to exercise, pick something you enjoy and will stick with. Start slow and commit to a doable amount of movement. Start with two or three sessions a week and stay there until you settle into a good, solid routine. Once you are in the groove, there you can eventually increase intensity, duration, and frequency if that is right for you.

Walking, running, cycling, weight training, climbing, swimming are all great options. Martial arts training and sparring, obstacle course training, functional movement exercises, boxing, cage fighting, and grappling are wonderful avenues for blowing off steam. If you aren't into the aggressive stuff, tai chi and **yoga** are calmer practices that have been around forever and can help you focus your mind, manage stress, boost health, increase vitality, and become less reactive.

After a back injury while lifting a 500lb patient, I was told I'd need surgery and pain pills for bulging discs. Instead of those options, I started doing yoga. Within a few weeks the pain went away and within a few months by back healed completely. No surgery needed.

While there are many branches, most styles incorporate movement with breath, teach you to become aware of the present moment, and get you back into your body. Don't worry—nobody is going to bend you into a pretzel right away. Instead, you can start with gentle classes that teach techniques and ease you into postures. By slowing down and connecting to our breath, we learn how to relax.

As a field, yoga is massive, with upwards of 14 types of yoga stemming from eight limbs. You don't need to understand the history of yoga in order to enjoy the benefits of practice. For more information, check out www.yogaforfirstresponders.org or visit a yoga studio near you.

Infrared Sauna

"Sitting in a infrared sauna three times a week helped my joint pain and muscle stiffness. I've had high blood pressure for a long time and that lowered after I started too."

– James, Homicide Detective

Unlike regular gym saunas, which heat you from the outside in, these saunas use infrared wavelengths to gently heat from the inside out. Infrared saunas are extremely popular in holistic healing communities due to their easy access, cost effectiveness, and powerful benefits including:

Pain Relief

Infrared heat relieves pain by expanding blood vessels and increasing circulation. This allows more oxygen to reach injured areas of the body, reducing pain and enhancing the healing process.

Immune System Support

The immune system weakens the hold of viruses and bacterial growth. Infrared heat induces a fever like signal by heating up the body but without the pains of an illness.

Elimination of Toxins

Sweating naturally rids the body of toxins but at a slow rate. Infrared heat stimulates the sweat glands to cleanse and detoxify at a higher rate.

Reduced Tension

Infrared heat loosens the muscles and relaxes the body. It naturally soothes the parasympathetic nervous system and signals the brain to induce a calm/healing state.

Cardiac Health

The heart receives a workout similar to a 6-mile run in a 20-30 minute infrared sauna session and produces a similar amount of sweat. Infrared saunas are perfect for those that do not have time for regular exercise or suffer from injuries that inhibit activity.

For more detailed information on infrared sauna benefits, check out www.sunlighten.com, or research where to find or buy an infrared sauna near you.

Establishing a New Identity

"I'm a medic and I suffer from PTSD, anxiety and depression. I'm on my journey to start a podcast that discusses these things and how the outdoors helps people heal. I have had lots of good feedback from my podcast and hunting community friends, and I will forever be trying to get rid of the stigma."

- Sarah Ann, Paramedic

Thinking about life beyond our current circumstance can be overwhelming when we are still drowning in our trauma. The thought of living in misery for another ten or twenty years can overtake us, and many people get beaten down, lose hope or give up.

I'm here to remind you that **just because it's been hard does not mean it always will be.** This entire book is dedicated to sharing the tools available for you to change your life. Sometimes, all we need is a bit of reassurance that it can be better, that healing beyond PTSD is possible.

Believe that a better life is possible.

If you have even the slightest hope that things can get better, that's enough. You don't have to know how to do it — you just need the willingness to try. If you don't believe that there is more for you, that's okay. Just apply the tools in this book and meet yourself where you are. REACH OUT to others for the support that you need until you do have a glimmer of hope. From there, you can begin the process of reconstructing a new identity beyond the trauma.

For many, establishing a new identity can be the most challenging aspect of all. Who are we if not the job? Who are we beyond the pain and trauma that we've experienced? What would life even be like if we were healthy, balanced and whole? Those are the powerful questions we must face in order to transform our suffering into wisdom.

Here are five modalities that can help you begin to form a new identity beyond PTSD:

Neuro-Linguistic Programming

"The job was my entire world — everything I'd ever wanted to be since I was a kid. So, when I retired out early, I had no idea what to do. It took a lot of rough years of drinking before I finally got help. My therapist and I did NLP together and it really helped. Within six months I started AA and eventually went back to school for my business degree. I finally see a light at the end of the tunnel."

– Jimmy, Firefighter

According to the NLP website: 'Neuro-Linguistic Programming is like a user's manual for the brain and taking an NLP training is like learning how to become fluent in the language of your mind so that the ever-so-helpful "server" that is your unconscious will finally understand what you actually want out of life. NLP is the study of excellent communication–both with yourself, and with others. NLP is a set of tools and techniques, but it is so much more than that. It is an attitude and a methodology of knowing how to achieve your goals and get results.' I've personally watched many people who have used NLP go on to become successful in business, finance, personal mastery and life. For more information visit www.nlp.com.

Intuitive Coaching

"Having a coach keeps me accountable to my goals. With her help, I found a purpose beyond 911 and went from rock bottom to up-and-running again in only a few months."

- Ryan, EMT

For many, figuring out what we want to do with our lives beyond a trauma can be incredibly challenging. In fact, it can be among the most challenging aspects of healing. It is for this this reason that working with a reputable intuitive healer or coach can help to bridge this gap. There are all kinds of healers out there, but what we want is someone who is grounded, well versed in trauma, and able to help you rebuild a new version of yourself. Having the guidance of another person can give you the courage to make the giant leap – and wow can it pay off! Rebuilding your life beyond the trauma or identity is no small feat! I highly recommend you seek the help of a coach to ease your transition. To find a coach/mentor near you, word of mouth is best. If you don't know anyone, check online, or reach out to me personally as I have helped countless first responders and military personnel from all over the world transform their lives. If you want holistic plan tailored specifically to you – hit me up. I'd be happy to help. www.sarahkgrace.com.

Visualization Techniques

"Believing is seeing and seeing is believing."

- Tom Hanks

We get so caught up in our history that it can be hard to fathom what life would be like any other way. This is where visualization comes in. The good news is that you can do this one alone — at least initially. Sitting down with a paper and pen, just start writing down things that you liked as a kid. Think about what you liked to do, what used to make you happy, or even what type of activity you would do for free now. Then move into any goals, dreams, or hopes that you have for your future. These remembrances begin the process of reconnecting you to a life beyond your current circumstance.

The ability to visualize your life beyond 'what was' plays a massive role in helping you to create it. In fact, visualizing, brainstorming, daydreaming, and daring to believe that you can create a new way of life is a cornerstone to healing beyond trauma. Believing that something new, different, and exciting is possible might sound lofty, but you'd be surprised just how quickly things change when you open to the possibility of new beginnings.

Try Something New

"Only those who will risk going too far can possibly find out how far one can go."

- T.S. Elliot

One great way to start building a life beyond trauma is by trying new things. Getting out of our everyday experience can bring fresh perspective and new ways of thinking about things. My absolute favorite way to do this is by traveling. Going places I've never been gets me out of my head and into the experience of living. We often get so stuck in our routine that we become prisoners to our experience — forgetting that there is a whole world out there beyond our little narrative. I've learned a lot about myself and other people when I get out of my little bubble to travel. You may have heard the saying, 'Sometimes we need to get lost to be found.' When we are willing to try new things, we bring in fresh perspective, opportunity and growth. These insights can offer us the glimmer of what's possible in life beyond our old trauma. If traveling isn't your thing, cool. Just write out a bucket list of experiences you've always wanted to have and start doing them. You'll be surprised at how much better you feel when you start living life instead of reacting to it.

Do Something You Think You Can't

"Whether you think you can or think you can't, you're right."

- Henry Ford

Most of us like a challenge, which is why we are first responders in the first place. We like to MacGyver our way through whatever craziness is around. This skillset can be used to our benefit when looking for a new role or identity by changing our narrative and introducing us to new ways of looking at things. Simply stated: when we do something we don't think we can do we gain self-confidence. That confidence can be built upon to form a new identity. Whether it's training for a Spartan race, learning to blacksmith, starting a non-profit that benefits soldiers or even writing a book about your own experiences — the process of challenging yourself and accomplishing a goal can be life changing to say the least.

"I have found that by doing new thing like going places I have never been, trying a sport I have never tried, eating different foods, changing it up and replacing the bad memories with new different ones has helped me the best. I am always scared for when symptoms will show up again but for now this is helping."

— Andrew, National Guard

Advice for Family Members

"The man I married is gone. I live with a stranger and don't know what to do anymore."

- Jenny, Wife of Marine Sergeant

Ali's Story

Jake and Ali were high school sweethearts with big dreams. Just after their wedding, Jake was hired onto the local fire department. Ali was over the moon to be married to a firefighter. She loved visiting the station and often spent hours making homemade cookies to bring to the crew.

The envy of her friends, she loved having a man in uniform and was proud to be a firefighter's wife. The first several years were a blissful whirlwind. Jake loved his job and promoted quickly within the department. The couple soon bought a quaint home and had two children. Everything was perfect! Ali stayed home with the kids, doting and nurturing them as Jake worked overtime to support the family financially.

The glow slowly started to fade, however, after series of fatal vehicle accident calls that Jake responded to. The carnage on those scenes haunted him and he slowly started to withdraw.

Ali noticed it, but she was so busy managing the kids, play dates, and chores that she thought it was just a phase. She figured they were trained for that kind of thing, and that he would eventually move through whatever it was he was dealing with. But Jake didn't move through it.

Weeks turned to months and he grew increasingly withdrawn from the family. Ali begged him repeatedly to talk to a counselor about was going on, but he couldn't yet cope with what he had seen, so instead of opening up to her, he shut her out. He started picking up more and more overtime and stayed at the station for days on end. When he did come home, he was snappy and tired. He spent most of his time sleeping or sitting in his recliner watching football, helping very little with the kids or anything around the house.

Another year passed and the once idyllic love of the two high school sweethearts soured. Overworked with kids and chores, Ali became bitterly resentful. She felt cheated. In her young naivety, she had believed that being married to a firefighter would be sexy and exciting—but now all she felt was baited, switched, and abandoned.

Jake worked constantly and she was left to raise the kids alone. He had become a vacant shell of the man she married. No longer fit and vibrant, he was lethargic, depressed, and withdrawn.

The couple regressed to screaming matches and door slamming. They argued for the sake of arguing, frightening the kids and wreaking havoc in the house. The deal breaker came when Ali tried to withdraw money at the bank but got an overdraft notice. After interrogating him, Jake finally broke down and told her that he had been secretly gambling. To her shock, he admitted to gambling away their entire savings and now their family home was on the line.

Ali lost it. She screamed bloody murder at Jake and wailed on him with her fists. Her heart was shattered.

She had tried so hard to be a good wife — to do everything right, but it had all gone to hell in a hand basket. The couple spent the next few months in half-hearted attempts at therapy for the sake of the children, but the damage had been done.

Ali eventually filed for divorce. She was bitter and heartbroken that her perfect life with a 'man in uniform' had become nothing less than a nightmare.

■

Family often gets caught in the crossfire of shift work, deployment, and PTSD. Divorce and broken homes are common among first responders and military due to the incredible strain duty can put on relationships.

Many military personnel and first responders often try to protect their spouses by not sharing the details of what they actually see and do at work. While those intentions may be good, that omission often leads to one partner feeling shut out.

The spouses I interviewed for this book relayed that they thought they knew what they were getting into when marrying a firefighter/police officer/soldier, etc. They really believed that they were strong enough to handle it. But as the years wore on, the isolation and instability got to be too much. Many I talked to fought hard and long to keep their marriage intact, but finally opted for divorce.

Here are the most frequent phrases used by spouses when interviewed for this book:

- I had no idea it would be this hard.
- The man/woman I married is completely different than who I live with now.
- Everything is on me: kids, cooking, bills, housework— everything.
- I'm exhausted.
- I'm scared that he will hurt/kill himself or hurt/kill me.
- I don't know how it got to be this bad.
- I am always walking on eggshells.
- I just want my husband back.
- I don't want to leave but I can't go on like this.
- We need help. We just don't know what to do.

PTSD support for those who have spent time on the front lines has become a hot topic in the mainstream media. While I'm happy that the discussion is finally happening, we don't hear as much about how difficult it can be on the families who live with those affected by PTSD. Very often, the spouse takes the brunt of it.

That is why I included this chapter— to **make sure the family members get their fair share of focus and support.** Living with and loving a person with PTSD can be very damaging to the family that is trying to support them, and I don't believe that is talked about enough. Very often, the spouse is left holding the bag: managing the children, chores, bills and responsibilities - all while navigating mood swings, outbursts, and flashbacks from their partner. It can be a lot to deal with. Sometimes it's too much.

Every situation is different. Some relationships last while others do not. What's most important is that the spouse of the person with PTSD prioritizes self care by keeping focus on their own health, wants, needs and capacity along the way. In some regards, being in relationship with a traumatized first responder is like being in relationship with an addict. The day to day experience can be irrational, unstable and exhausting if you don't take measure to put yourself and your children first.

Caregiver burnout is common when dealing with years of PTSD cycles. If this describes you, here are some factors to consider for the long haul:

Try not to take it personally. Easier said than done, I know, but wounded people wound people. Your partner's behavior likely has more to do with their own issues than it does you. By trying to not taking things personally, you can create a buffer so that you don't shoulder responsibility for things that are not yours to carry.

Find support. This is essential for your overall longevity and wellbeing. Having friends, family, or a support network of people who understand your situation and can offer respite is critical. Trying to 'go it alone' is noble, but not sustainable. It's not possible to carry this heavy of a burden on your own. Your body and mind will break down from the pressure.

Reach out. Ask for help. I cannot emphasize enough how critical this is. If you don't have anyone physically close to you, online groups can be a great way to connect with other like-minded people around the world. Having the right support can be the pivotal factor in the survivability of your relationship.

Know your limits. Sometimes we give away too much of ourselves in order to make things work. Beware of martyr syndrome– putting everyone else's needs first- to your own detriment. I advocate that you have compassion for your spouse's process, but retain your own personal power. Partnership is a two-party deal. Too often one person assumes all the responsibility and holds up the entire relationship. That's not fair or sustainable. Additionally, gauge your partner's willingness to get help and change. If they are open to helping themselves, there is hope that things can get better. If they are not, take an honest look at that. Unwillingness to seek help or take personal responsibility by one party often means that things will not only stay the same, but could actually get worse.

Ask yourself: How much more of this can I handle? What are *my* needs? Are they being met? What can I do today to help myself? You matter too. Have the courage to put yourself first so that you have the energy to stay balanced. Lastly, if you are attacked, threatened or assaulted I urge you to seek immediate counseling and/or remove yourself and your children from the situation.

Here are some questions for the family to consider for their healing process:

- Am I happy in my life/relationship?
- What is working? What isn't?
- What do I love most about my spouse?
- Why do I stay?
- What are the most challenging aspects of our dynamic?
- Do I feel safe?
- Do I feel loved?
- Am I appreciated?
- What can I do to make my own situation better?
- What do I want/need?
- What is my vision for my life?
- Is he/she willing to change?
- Am I willing to change?
- Who or what is my support system?
- What can I do today to change myself for the better?

"Being married to a combat vet has been very challenging, and at the same time very rewarding. He is gone a lot, so I make sure to keep myself engaged in my own life and goals. By keeping the focus on myself first, I am able to stay happy and focused on making my life and relationship how I want it to be."

- Susan, Wife of Army Officer

Craig's Story

Craig spent twenty years active duty in the Marine Corps – Forces Special Operations Command. With seven long, violent tours under his belt he was notorious throughout the ranks for his leadership and incredible combat skills. He was 'the man' and everyone wanted to have him on their side during a fire fight.

After retiring though, Craig began having a very difficult time coping with civilian life. His wife brought him into my office for a session with me after she found him in a PTSD flashback - standing at full attention on the lawn in his underwear at dawn with his gun locked and loaded by his side. He had no idea how he had gotten there. Frightened, she called out to snap him back to reality as she had done so many times before. Fortunately, they had been doing counseling together and this method worked for them. Craig 'woke up' out of his PTSD trance before any violence ensued. He had no recollection of grabbing his gun or walking outside. That level of disassociation scared him.

Craig didn't understand how he could black out but still be up moving around. It really scared him for and he decided to get help for the sake of his wife and kids. While in session, we chatted about trauma and the brain before working together to formulate a 'treatment plan', which included grounding exercises, breathing techniques, energy work, acupuncture, Chinese herbs, and EMDR. We also devised a plan to secure his firearms and get his entire family counseling. His wife also decided to join a codependent group where she was able to find support with her challenges. Six weeks later Craig stopped by my office to share his progress...

He hadn't had a flashback since starting his program and his home life was less volatile. While they all still had a lot of work to do to get stabilized, Craig and his family had taken giant first steps towards a healthier future.

Real Talk About Suicide

"I can't do it anymore. I know how I'm going to go; I'm just trying to get the courage. I'm tired of thinking that I'm going to get better and then collapsing again. It'll be better for those around me in the long run."

- **Dustin, US Navy Veteran**

Suicide has become one of the leading causes of death for front line workers.
It's time we talk about it.

We are living in an unprecedented time where first responders are more likely to die by suicide than in the line of duty. Think about that for a minute... So many of us are hurting so badly that we are ending our own lives in droves. The past few years have shown a marked increase in military and first responder suicides as well as workplace violence.

Are you at your breaking point? Are you past it?

If so, you are not alone. I've worked with suicidal first responders and military personnel and do you know what I've learned? Most of them really don't want to die — they just want the pain to stop.

Can you relate?

How would your life be different if you had the tools to deal with all of that you have seen and experienced?

It is clear that we are at a crisis level and that action is required. Suicide has always occurred to varying degrees in our field, but the evolution of the internet combined with the brave men and women coming forward to talk openly about their PTSD has made us even more aware of its pervasiveness. While open dialogue is great, there are still two primary obstacles that prevent many people from getting the help they need:

1) Stigma. This is likely a primary force behind keeping us from getting the help we need. Nobody wants to be 'that guy' – you know, the one who can't "handle it." So, we quietly stuff it all down and slowly degrade until we either change or break.

Unfortunately, we've lost countless personnel to addiction and suicide over the years as a result of this stigma. The glimmer of hope is that we are now becoming aware of the magnitude of the problem and positive changes are beginning to take place. Help is on the way.

2) Willingness to help others but unwillingness to help ourselves. I can't tell you how often I see this. Many front line workers have the tools and resources at their disposal, but they just won't use them to help themselves.

It seems that people with this personality type often have a much easier time rescuing others than they do themselves. For whatever reason (family dynamics, childhood instability, guilt, fear, etc.) the individual is often much more comfortable prioritizing other people's needs ahead of their own - sometimes to their own peril.

While these obstacles definitely exist, they do not have to prevent you from getting the help you need! Fortunately, more resources are becoming available as more and more people talk openly about their battles with PTSD.

YOU ARE NOT ALONE.

YOU DO NOT HAVE TO CARRY THIS BY YOURSELF ANY LONGER.

IT'S OKAY TO ASK FOR HELP.

A good first step in suicide prevention is acknowledging that you are not okay.

This takes courage and can be harder than we realize for those in our profession. Like we covered in earlier chapters, the first responder archetype is one of heroics and external intensity. Admitting that we are struggling goes against that grain. That internal discord can really become an issue as we keep living, working, and pretending like everything is fine. Truly, though – nothing will change as long as we avoid what is really going on within us. In fact, it will likely only get worse.

Please understand that times are changing. Acceptance and openness are replacing the old 'suck it up' mentality. People all over are beginning to realize the extreme toll a life of service can have on a person and their family – and fortunately, programs are being developed and put into curriculum to combat the heaviness.

Being depressed, anxious, overwhelmed or even suicidal doesn't make you less of a person… in fact, the depths of those emotions demonstrate your humanity.

It's okay to not be strong all the time.

Some of the bravest people I've ever known were warriors on the front lines and then came home to battle their inner demons head on.

"I measure success one day at a time. After many years my suicidal ideation is under control. I've had a good experience with the VA, some bumps in the road, but overall good. I've dumped my bag or rocks and replaced it with my "life bag." In there I put good experiences. We have to give ourselves permission to find some enjoyment in every day. I often have to remind myself that I am my harshest critic, and when I'm able to do that, it is a good experience."

- Jonathan, Veteran

Some Statistics About Suicide:

- There are currently between 25-35 first responder and military personnel suicides every day.

- Many more go unreported.

- Addiction often contributes to premature death and/or suicide.

- Alcoholism is the #1 reported coping mechanism for first responders.

- Workplace violence and on duty death/suicides have escalated significantly in the last decade.

- First responder/military suicide is often impulsive and not planned out.

- The deadly triad: depression, alcohol and a firearm.

- Studies show people who actually follow through on completing suicide think about it for only five minutes before acting.

If you are contemplating suicide, here are three things you can do to immediately help yourself:

1. **Reach out.** Tell someone – anyone – about your experience.

2. **Resist the impulse to self-harm.** You can do this by breathing deeply, moving your body, and getting yourself out of isolation.

3. **Find a friend or licensed trauma therapist** who can help you process and get you equipped with a plan.

My brother is a police officer and over the course of his career, I watched him go downhill with his stress and PTSD. Initially, he didn't seem that bad since he was always the strong one. He held everything together for the family - especially around his kids, but inside he was really suffering. When he ended up in the hospital after a suicide attempt, we were all shocked. I guess he just didn't know how to ask for help. Later he said that he felt like a burden and just didn't want to feel that pain any more. It has been a long road, but he's in therapy now and even tried some yoga classes with me recently. We talk more and I feel closer to him now than I ever did growing up. After what happened, I needed support, too – I had so much guilt. But we're slowly taking steps toward healing. Sometimes it's so hard to trust the process, but it's getting better every day.
- Hannah, Sister of Lieutenant

I never wanted to let other people think I was weak, but inside I was losing it. Life was just getting worse and worse. Suicidal thoughts. Panic attacks. Drinking to blackout. Fights with my wife. I'm glad now that I didn't take action to kill myself, but I sure didn't feel like living another day. That was rock bottom for me.
- John, Battalion Chief

You are worth it.

Your life is worth living.

This moment will pass.

If you have been looking for a sign to live, this is it.

National Suicide Prevention Hotline:
800-273-8255

Crisis Text Line:
Text HELLO to 741741

The National Suicide Prevention Lifeline is a national network of local crisis centers that provides free and confidential emotional support to people in suicidal crisis or emotional distress 24 hours a day, 7 days a week. All calls are confidential.

Signs and Symptoms[1]

The behaviors listed below may be signs that someone is thinking about suicide.

- Talking about wanting to die or wanting to kill themselves
- Talking about feeling empty, hopeless, or having no reason to live
- Making a plan or looking for a way to kill themselves, such as searching for lethal methods online, stockpiling pills, or buying a gun
- Talking about great guilt or shame
- Talking about feeling trapped or feeling that there are no solutions
- Feeling unbearable pain (emotional pain or physical pain)
- Talking about being a burden to others
- Using alcohol or drugs more often
- Acting anxious or agitated
- Withdrawing from family and friends
- Changing eating and/or sleeping habits
- Showing rage or talking about seeking revenge
- Taking great risks that could lead to death, such as driving extremely fast
- Talking or thinking about death often
- Displaying extreme mood swings, suddenly changing from very sad to very calm or happy
- Giving away important possessions
- Saying goodbye to friends and family
- Putting affairs in order, making a will

---

[1] From the National Institute of Mental Health:
https://www.nimh.nih.gov/health/topics/suicide-prevention/

If these warning signs apply to you or someone you know, get help as soon as possible, particularly if the behavior is new or has increased recently.

How to Help[2]

If someone you know is struggling, here are 5 action steps for helping someone in emotional pain.

ASK: "Are you thinking about killing yourself?" It's not an easy question, but studies show that asking at-risk individuals if they are suicidal does not increase suicides or suicidal thoughts.

KEEP THEM SAFE: Reducing a suicidal person's access to highly lethal items or places is an important part of suicide prevention. While this is not always easy, asking if the at-risk person has a plan and removing or disabling the lethal means can make a difference.

---

[2] From the National Institute of Mental Health: https://www.nimh.nih.gov/health/topics/suicide-prevention/

BE THERE: Listen carefully and learn what the individual is thinking and feeling. Research suggests acknowledging and talking about suicide may reduce rather than increase suicidal thoughts.

HELP THEM CONNECT: Save the National Suicide Prevention Lifeline's (1-800-273-TALK (8255)) and the Crisis Text Line's number (741741) in your phone, so it's there when you need it. You can also help make a connection with a trusted individual like a family member, friend, spiritual advisor, or mental health professional.

STAY CONNECTED: Staying in touch after a crisis or after being discharged from care can make a difference. Studies have shown the number of suicide deaths goes down when someone follows up with the at-risk person.

Lindsay's Story

Lindsay was an EMT in Oakland. Shaken after the traumatic death of a close family member, she nevertheless decided to push through by going back to work as soon as possible after the funeral. At first, she was fine but she became increasingly aggravated on calls, especially CPR's and car accidents.

Within a few months her symptoms increased to the point that she froze at the very thought of responding to a trauma call. Lindsay eventually became very angry and "not a nice person to be around." Before she was diagnosed with PTSD, she took out all of that anger on her partner, who had been trying patiently to help her for months.

Defiant, Lindsay refused anyone's advice or help. Eventually other coworkers complained about her negative behavior. Some were worried about her while others were just tired of dealing with her poor attitude on scene. A division manager pulled Lindsay aside one day and had a very frank conversation. He said that her behavior was beginning to affect her work and that he recommended she take some time off.

During the time at home, things got really bad for Lindsay. Her anxiety and depression skyrocketed and she had vivid nightmares about car accidents and dead bodies every night. After one particularly upsetting dream, Lindsay decided that she didn't want to live anymore. She hastily wrote a suicide note and grabbed her gun. Just as she was about to pull the trigger, the phone rang. It was her good friend and supervisor who said, "I just had a feeling I needed to check up on you. Are you alright?"

That moment changed everything. Taking it as a sign that it wasn't her time to die, Lindsay finally decided to get help. She was put in touch with a therapist who practiced EMDR. Skeptical at first, Lindsay didn't feel like anything was happening. But eventually the more she opened up, the better she started to feel. Realizing that her anger had ruined many friendships and relationships throughout her life, she took ownership of her past behaviors and made amends with the people she had hurt. With her therapist's support, she got to the root of her traumas and slowly took charge of her health. She cut back on junk food and alcohol, started walking every day, and got a service dog named Harley who helped tremendously with his constant support.

It's been a long road for Lindsay, but today she is happier than she's been in a long time. Back at work, she now is an advocate for her coworkers to reach out for help when they need it. She shares openly about her experience and promotes the benefits service animals throughout many local and state agencies. Lindsay leads by example that self-care, ownership, and willingness to change is imperative to a lasting career as a first responder.

Conclusion

Congratulations on almost completing this book! My hope is that you found some of the stories and tools relatable and inspiring. There is a lot of information listed here, and I encourage you to take your recovery process one day at a time. Healing doesn't happen overnight, but big changes can happen by making small changes every day.

You – and your family – are worth it.

∎

As a bonus, I put some of the thought provoking questions from the Holistic PTSD Recovery Workbook in the last section of this book. Read them over. Ponder. Maybe even grab a pen and paper and write down your answers. The deeper you are willing to go into your process – the faster your healing can happen.

∎

You are my brothers and sisters.

I want honor you for all that you are, and all that you have been through.

Please don't give up. Even in your darkest hour, know that you are not alone. You have what it takes to pull through.

It's finally your turn to feel good again. And now, you have the tools to do just that. Are you ready?

HOLISTIC PTSD RECOVERY RECAP

Find what works for you.

Restore Biochemistry of the Brain
Brainspotting / EMDR
Binaural Audio
Biofeedback
Hypnotherapy
Breathing Techniques

Release Trauma from the Body
Craniosacral Therapy
Trauma Release Exercises (TRE)
Float Tanks
Myofascial Release
Reiki

Process Difficult Emotions
Somatic Trauma Therapy
Meditation
Acupuncture
Journaling
Rage Release Exercises

Reclaim Physical Health
Nutrition
Hydration
Sleep Exercise
Infrared Sauna

Establish a New Identity
Neurolinguistic Programming (NLP)
Intuitive Coaching
Visualization Techniques
Try Something New
Do Something You Think You Can't

HOLISTIC PTSD RECOVERY WORKBOOK SAMPLE

Below are a few sample questions from the Holistic PTSD Recovery Workbook. They are designed to get you actively participating in your healing process. The workbook offers even more questions and space to write out your answers and reflect in more detail. It's available on Amazon or my website, along with helpful audio meditations and an herbal blend for PTSD if you are interested in additional tools for support.

Basics

- How did you come to be a first responder or in the military?
- Did you grow up wanting to do it?
- Has your career been what you thought it would be? Explain.
- What is your favorite part of your job?
- What is your least favorite?

Coping

- My PTSD symptoms are:
- My top PTSD triggers are:
- On a scale of 1-10 my typical stress level is:
- How well do I handle my stress?
- What part of my life is most stressful?
- What is the second most stressful part of my life?
- How do I cope? (exercise, drinking, gambling, etc.)

Willingness

- I am open to change: True / False
- I am willing to be accountable for my life: True / False
- I am open to asking for help when I need it: True / False
- I am willing to consider other people's opinions: True / False
- I am willing to surrender control: True / False
- I am always right: True / False

Physical

- I have pain in my body: True / False
- I have headaches and neck tension: True / False
- I have back problems: True / False
- I clench my jaw or grind my teeth: True /
- True / False
- I sleep well and feel rested: True / False
- I take good care of my physical body: True / False
- I eat a healthy diet: True / False
- I drink enough water: True / False
- What are three positive changes I could make to become healthier?
- Am I willing to view things in my life differently?
- How do I let my anger get the better of
- Do I believe that healing is possible?
- What would my life be like if I was healed from PTSD?
- My ideal life looks like:

Family

- Do I feel close to my immediate family?
- Is it easy or hard for me to talk to them? Why or why not?
- Do I feel understood by my family? Why or why not?
- Do I feel supported by my family? Why or why not?
- Is it hard for me to let my guard down and get close to others? If so, why?
- Do I have good communication with my family? Why or why not?
- How could I be a better communicator?
- Do I consider my family's needs in addition to my own?
- Do I prioritize my family?
- Am I willing to hear my partner's feelings? Why or why not?
- Am I sensitive to my partner's needs? Why or why not?
- How would my family describe me?
- Am I willing to take ownership of my faults?
- Do I realize that nobody can change me but me?
- Am I willing to change?

Personal Experience

Next, we will delve into some of the events that may have contributed greatly to your PTSD. Please take this section slowly.

If you become triggered, take a break. Take a few deep breaths, go for a walk outside or jump in a cool shower and wait until the symptoms subside before continuing.

If these questions are too much, find someone that you trust and/or professional help to help you work through them. The only way out is through. That said you don't have to do this alone. Therapists, healers, mentors, trusted officers and superiors are great allies when facing the tough triggers and symptoms of trauma.

- My worst 911 call, deployment, or tour ever was:
- What bothered me most about it?
- If you can, write out in details that challenge you the most from the call/tour.
- How does my body react when I think about it?
- Are there areas of tightness, pressure or pain? If so, feel the sensations of the body and very gently allow them to surface. Take a few deep breaths as they arise and allow the sensation to pass. Trust that you can handle it.

- What happens in my mind when I think about that call/tour? Does it spin out? Flashback? If your mind races or PTSD cascade begins, clap your hands together then *gently* slap all over your arms, legs, and body. This can help bring you back into the present moment and dissipate symptoms.

- How has this call/tour impacted me?
- What PTSD symptoms do I have as a result?
- What triggers these symptoms in my everyday life?
- Am I willing to get professional help?
- Do I believe that I can be free of my PTSD?
- Am I willing to face my fears?
- Am I willing to tackle my addictions?
- What would my life be like if I was healed from my PTSD?
- What are three things I need to change in order to heal myself?
- Am I ready to make those changes?

You've reached the end of this book—*well done!*

My hope is that the tools and information provided here will support you as you continue your life and career. Whether you are new to your role, continuing your years of service, or you have already retired, it's never too early or too late to do this work.

The healing process can be a slow and sometimes arduous journey and my guess is that this book brought up a lot for you. If that's the case, please know that you are on the right track. If you need help, reach out to me or to any of the amazing resources listed in this book.

Take it one day at a time.

Healing happens in stages – not overnight.

Even though it may not always feel it, your efforts in this world matter.

You matter.

I celebrate the great gift you have given yourself by embarking on your healing journey.

From one to another, thank you for all that you do.

I see you. I honor you. And I believe in you.

"I wish all victims of PTSD in the Military would come to understand that they are precious to us. That there is nothing wrong with you, there is something right about you! It's a normal response to something wrong (war) and you aren't weak, just a little bit broken. You can and will survive. You will feel love and feel "normal" again through family or community help and support. Get help, reach out, don't hold back...tell a friend, your family, a doctor, a therapist. Reach out! Please! You are worth it!"

- Kevin, father of a veteran with PTSD

About the Author

Sarah K. Grace is a powerful and dynamic individual who spent nearly two decades merging her career as a paramedic in some of California's busiest 911 systems with her innate gifts as a medical intuitive and clairvoyant healer. Combining Western and Energy Medicine, Sarah spent years studying both physical and energy anatomy while applying her skills in critical settings to thousands of patients as they dealt with life and death emergencies.

Sarah is now a sought-after author, speaker, and healer who bridges western medicine with holistic healing. She teaches people how to heal the root of their trauma by providing step-by-step guidance and powerful healing sessions. Sarah has worked with thousands of first responders and other people worldwide as they integrate PTSD, overcome addiction, rediscover their personal power, and step into their intuitive gifts.

Sarah is a vibrant person who employs quick wit and dry humor to connect with her clients. She pulls from her own experience to lead by example that full recovery from trauma and addiction is not only possible, but also that intuitive gifts can be the key to an extraordinary life.

To connect with Sarah or to book a session, visit www.sarahkgrace.com.